OUTLIERS

— IN —

MEDICINE

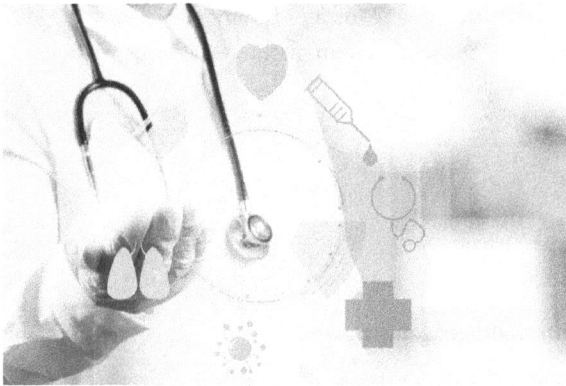

BY JOHN SHUFELDT

Inquiries should be addressed to:
Outliers Publishing
Hangar 1
7332 E. Butherus Drive
Scottsdale, AZ 85260

info@ingredientsofoutliers.com

ISBN: 978-1-940288-10-9

Cover design by paja-o@live.com

Interior production by Perfect Bound Marketing + Press, Inc.

Manuscript review by Bob Kelly of WordCrafters, Inc.

TABLE OF CONTENTS

Introduction v

Chapter 1 | Dr. Robin Blackstone 1

Chapter 2 | Dr. Robert Cromer 19

Chapter 3 | Dr. Matthew Hummel 33

Chapter 4 | Jessie Kiljonen. 47

Chapter 5 | Dr. Rachel Lindor. 59

Chapter 6 | Dr. Angela Nuzzarello 75

Resources 85

Conclusion. 99

Additional Works by Dr. John Shufeldt 101

INTRODUCTION

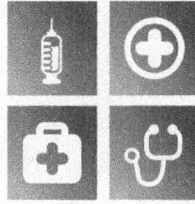

*"The practice of medicine is an art, not a trade;
a calling, not a business; a calling in which your heart
will be exercised equally with your head."*

~ Sir William Osler

The healthcare delivery system has changed a lot since I became a doctor in 1986. Back then, there were far fewer professional directions from which to choose. After completing medical school and your residency, you could decide to enter practice or subspecialize. You could start your own practice, work in a hospital, or work in research and education.

Today, with the onset of medical innovation and technological developments, you have the ability to reach patients in remote areas and outside of office hours through telemedicine. Or bring lifesaving vaccines to a third world country in a "smart" fridge, one that keeps track of inventory and sends data when more supplies are needed. Your patients will be able to send you their vitals through a wearable device that help you better monitor and manage their health. You have even more unique opportunities in front of you that we can't even imagine today.

Your decision to pursue medicine will mean a long road ahead of you, of challenging exams, grueling hours, and years of postgraduate studies.

It's critical that you know your options and perform as many informational interviews as you can. So I invited a few of my colleagues in various stages of their careers to "sit down" and share their professional experiences with you. You'll hear from:

- an industry leading bariatric surgeon whose passion for her patients and her focus on her discipline will inspire and energize you;

- a private practice owner with a full spectrum of services;

- a medical school student who offers tips for getting the most out of your undergraduate degree;

- an emergency medicine physician who offers advice about choosing a school and career path;

- an accomplished and dynamic medical educator whose focus is on the career development and wellness of medical students and physicians;

- And an old-school family physician who has since passed away, leaving his final words with us about his passion for medicine and some true tales about running a family practice.

I hope their stories are not only inspiring, but help you decide whether practicing medicine is for you, and which professional direction excites you.

But before I "hand over the microphone," so to speak, let's talk more about the future of healthcare you're stepping into.

Today, in virtually every industry and every profession, technology-driven disruption has been the topic of the day, nationally as well as globally. That's certainly the case in the medical profession. Such tools as artificial intelligence, virtual reality, robotics, and machine learning are changing the way doctors and their patients interact. While such routine tasks as record-keeping and appointments are easily automated, there has been considerable debate about the coming scope of healthcare in general and of tomorrow's doctors in particular.

In the latter case, speculation has varied widely, from gradually diminishing roles to significantly expanding ones, with the latter position greatly outweighing the former. Among the most popular views is that the impact of technology on various occupations will be much less than on specific activities within those occupations, while redefining specific roles and processes.

The prestigious global management consulting firm, McKinsey & Company, issued a preliminary report on an extensive study it conducted, confirming that view. The report also noted that "even the highest-paid *occupations* in the economy, such as financial managers, physicians, and senior executives, including CEOs, have a significant amount of activity that can be automated."

In a recent blog post, physician and author Bertalan Mesko, of the Medical Futurist Institute, wrote: "Artificial narrow intelligence (ANI) will most likely help healthcare move from traditional, "one-size-fits-all" medical solutions toward targeted treatments, personalized therapies, and uniquely composed drugs. In two words: precision medicine."

As a physician, I'm excited about what lies ahead in our profession, and I tend to believe that, were he alive today, Sir William Osler, whom I quoted above, would share in that excitement as well. Let me explain why.

In 1872, Canadian-born William Osler received his medical degree from McGill University in Montreal. After postgraduate studies abroad, he returned to Canada in 1874 and joined the McGill faculty. In 1884, he left to become professor of clinical medicine at the University of Pennsylvania.

Known for his innovative approach to treating patients, his reputation grew rapidly and, in 1888, he was recruited to become physician-in-chief of the soon to be opened Johns Hopkins Hospital in Baltimore and as professor of medicine of its planned school of medicine. To this day, Osler is recognized as one of the fathers of modern medicine.

Among his many accomplishments, Osler was the first physician to bring his medical students out of the classroom for training right at the bedside of patients. Often described as among "the greatest diagnosticians ever to wield a stethoscope," he created the first residency program to train specialists. In 1892, his book, *The Principles and Practice of Medicine*, was published, and would remain among the most significant medical textbooks for 40 years.

I'm confident Doctor Osler would feel right at home among the six professionals whose stories follow.

CHAPTER 1

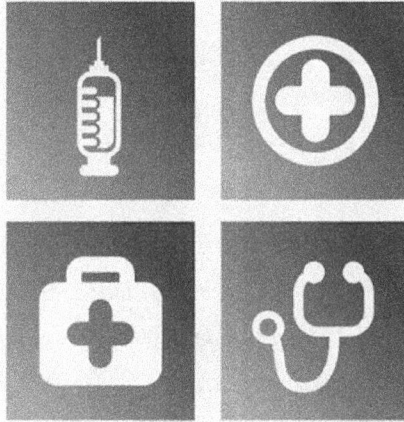

Dr. Robin Blackstone

BIOGRAPHY

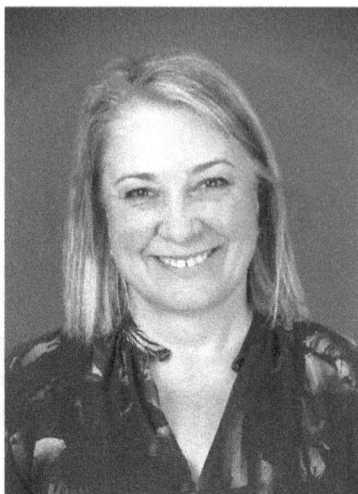

"Even at times when I've had really hard times, like there is nothing quite as difficult as working as a surgery resident... But remember that if you choose to quit, it will last a whole lifetime... So, whatever you're going through at that moment, if you can just figure out a way to get to the next moment and through that little patch, remember that things will change, they will improve, you'll sleep more, and they'll be better. You'll look back on it and realize that if you had quit it would have been the biggest mistake you'd ever made."

- Dr. Robin Blackstone

Dr. Robin Blackstone is a nationally recognized bariatric surgeon and bariatric medicine specialist who directs the Center for Obesity and Bariatric Surgery at Banner University Medical Center in Phoenix, Arizona. Recognized as a leading expert in the field of surgical treatment of obesity and obesity related diseases, she has dedicated her practice and career to improving the health of people affected by obesity. She is committed to advocacy for quality of life for the obese, and to establishing effective programs for the safe care of patients with obesity that span the medical and surgical continuum.

Dr. Blackstone graduated from the University of Texas Medical School at San Antonio and has performed more than 7,000 bariatric surgeries since she transitioned from surgical oncology to bariatric surgery in 2001. In addition, she is a Professor of Surgery at the University of Arizona College of Medicine – Phoenix, and served as the first woman president of the American Society for Metabolic and Bariatric Surgery.

A passionate teacher of surgery residents and medical students, she has directed a dynamic week-long course, "Obesity Week," for the second-year medical students annually for the last 11 years at UA Phoenix. She is a champion of gender equality for pay and promotions in academic medicine, mentoring many men and women in medicine.

Dr. Blackstone has received many awards throughout her career. In 2004, she was named to the American College of Surgeons National Faculty in Bariatric Surgery. Since 2005, after rigorous application and review, her surgery practice has repeatedly earned the highly prized recognition as a nationally accredited center by the American College of Surgeons. In 2017, she was awarded the ASMBS LEAD award for Quality and Patient Safety.

Dr. Blackstone is a founding board member of the Obesity Action Coalition, a national group dedicated to both promoting access to care for obesity and raising awareness of obesity discrimination. She also serves as a governor of the American College of Surgeons and is a past president of the North American Chapter of the International Federation of Obesity.

She is the author/editor of numerous books, book chapters and peer reviewed articles on obesity medicine, metabolic surgery and patient safety and quality. She single-authored the premier medical treatise, *Obesity: The Medical Practitioner's Essential Guide*, published in 2016.

She also served as editor of the comprehensive surgery textbook, *The ASMBS Textbook of Bariatric Surgery*, published in 2015.

Dr. Blackstone's most recent professional project outside the operating theater is a collaborative effort with the Harvard School of Business to create a Time Drive, Activity Based Costing Model for Obesity surgery, with the goal of developing a global population management program for patients suffering from obesity.

INTERVIEW

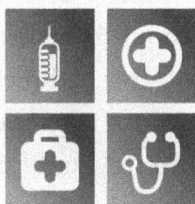

Q: When did you know you wanted to be a doctor?

A: I grew up in the Grand Canyon National Park, and there weren't a lot of professional people around. We didn't have a hospital, but we did have a doctor who had an urgent care clinic. When I was five, I'd torn some ligaments in my foot trying to learn to ski, and I remember this doctor taking care of me. I wrote in my school yearbook that I wanted to be a doctor after this.

That doctor was a central figure in the Grand Canyon National Park. I remember him as one of those people everyone relied on. If you needed to turn to him for help, you'd get help. Being a healer, or being someone who plays that role, was important to me. Throughout my life, in most of my relationships, I've played something of that role with people: friends, coworkers, and certainly with my patients.

There's a precedent in my family in healthcare as well. My great-grandmother practiced folk medicine, and my grandmother was a nurse's aide in the hospital in Jerome, Arizona and later in Prescott, Arizona. When I was in high school, I worked during one summer at night as a nurse's aide and the following summer at the Veterans Administration. These early experiences lent strength to the decision I'd made about becoming a physician.

Q: How did you find your way to medicine?

A: For awhile, I did other things. When I graduated from college with my degree in philosophy, I realized I didn't really have a skill I could get a job with. I also had met Al Staerkel, who became my husband over that summer after graduating from college. I worked in an insurance office as a secretary, and I can still remember thinking to myself, "This is absolutely not going to continue. I mean, I hate myself." If I hate something, then I change it!

Eventually, I realized I wanted to be a doctor. So, I ended up back in school at Houston Baptist University. There was a woman there named Dr. Joyce Fan; she was someone you could go to who'd help you analyze whether or not you could get to be a doctor. I told her my story. Even though I only had a philosophy degree from college, I said, "I want to go to medical school and become a physician."

She said, "Well, let's see if you have an aptitude. I want you to take organic chemistry this summer." With no other preamble, I jumped into this organic chemistry class that she taught. At the end of the summer, I'd taken both semesters and only missed one point. So she said, "You know what, I think you can work hard enough and I think you have the aptitude."

I went ahead and got all my prerequisites and was accepted into medical school at the University of Texas in San Antonio. Then, of course, I fell in love with surgery.

Q: Why did you fall in love with surgery?

A: When I grew up in the Grand Canyon, I had to sew many of my own clothes. My mother taught me to sew and after I had mastered the basics, I gravitated toward the complex patterns instead of the simple ones because I liked the intricacy of design. Surgery is similar to sewing clothes, in that it requires both strategic and tactical skills.

There was something about the focus and the intensity of surgery that really spoke to me.

Q: How did you decide on bariatric surgery?

A: My practice of surgery up until 2000 was primarily centered in surgical oncology. I also did very advanced general surgery procedures with the laparoscope. During an especially stressful time, I became overwhelmed by emotion and felt I needed to take a serious break and think about the kind of medicine I was practicing. I closed my practice in oncology in September of 2000 and took the next nine months off. During that time, I did some traveling, and when a local bariatric surgeon asked me to help him learn a laparoscopic gastric bypass, I went back to the OR and after a few cases I was really intrigued by this new specialty that was emerging in treating obese patients. A survey of the national landscape showed there were few truly excellent centers for treatment.

When I established the Scottsdale Bariatric Center, I designed it to try to put together a comprehensive treatment plan for people who suffer from obesity and its related medical problems.

That's where I found my stride, in a sense, because it was a group of people against whom it's still okay to be prejudiced and treat them with disrespect – I hated that. They couldn't get access to the procedures that could help fix a lot of the medical problems they had. They were invisible to the medical profession, who had little scientific background to understand the truth about obesity, and didn't know how to help them. It totally captured my imagination and ignited within me a drive to help.

Scottsdale Bariatric Center was established and started to provide surgical treatment of obesity in November of 2001. Since that time my assistant, Melissa Davis, DNP and I have operated on and cared for more than 5,000 people suffering from morbid obesity.

Q: Do you also teach?

A: I'm grateful for being able to try and communicate what I know in a way that makes it useful to others. We have such a dynamic and rich clinical setting that having medical students, nurse practitioner students and residents work with our team is an honor. Our team also conducts a week-long course called "Obesity Week," at the University of Arizona School of Medicine-Phoenix.

Perhaps our most important teaching is through our public education seminars that are given weekly and available online to teach people who suffer from obesity the science of the disease and its consequences and really give them options that relate to their lives and may help them work through obesity to better health.

Q: Was passion important in your pursuit and in your life?

A: Passion has driven most of my life. When I attempt to engage anything, it's the romance of it that grabs me. Surgery is certainly like that.

When I was at Houston Baptist University, one of my peers in my physics class who was a scrub-tech said to me, "Why don't you come and watch surgery? I can get you in."

I said, "Okay." It turned out she worked at Baylor School of Medicine and was the personal scrub tech to Michael E. DeBakey, the heart surgeon. I arrived before dawn and was privileged to watch him and his team for an entire day. I was still standing there watching my third heart operation long after the sun had set.

I remember Dr. DeBakey, who hadn't talked to me all day, say, "Don't you have a home to go to?"

I said, "Maybe, but I don't remember that right now." Seeing him walk down the hall, with his white coat flowing behind him, and thinking about the impact of his life on others, was such a romantic notion. Surgery is very dramatic.

Passion for surgery and the care of patients is very strong in me. I love taking things on that are hard to learn, complex or hard to do, and when you do them it seems as if your whole soul is engaged in it. If I don't feel that way about something, I tend not to pick it up or try it.

Q: When you first starting pursuing medicine, were you apprehensive about it?

A: Most of the time, I don't use or recognize the word or feeling of apprehension. I'm one of these people who, if you give me a challenge, I'll find some way to meet it. I've been like that my whole life. That's just me. Medical school was a challenge. I just had to figure out how to meet it.

For example, in college, I had to take calculus. You have to take it to get into medical school. It's kind of crazy because calculus is irrelevant to medicine in most ways in which you practice as a physician. But, it's relevant in terms of critical thinking.

Well, the thing about calculus was that I needed to earn an "A." My husband felt that, if I couldn't do that in these prerequisite courses, I needed to abandon my goal of being a physician and have a child. In my mind, a "B" meant "Baby." Not that I was opposed to having kids, but I didn't feel I'd be able to take on both being a mother and trying to pursue medicine.

On my first calculus test, I earned 89 percent. Mathematically, it's hard to recover from that because an "A" grade required 93 percent or higher. So I went to the professor, to ask how I might reach that goal.

He said, "You thought through the calculus perfectly, but you can't add a column of numbers and come out with the right amount. Every problem you missed was due to the algebra, not the calculus."

I said, "Well what can I do about it?"

He took this old, dusty book from his bookshelf, handed it to me and said, "Do the problems in here and I'll grade every one of them."

I came back a few days later and had five chapters done. I handed him this huge stack of paper. He said, "You're really serious about this."

I said, "I have to do what I can do. If I don't earn an "A" but try my hardest, that's fine. But it's not going to be because I didn't do everything I could."

They posted final grades in those days, and so my husband and I drove over there. I remember getting out of the car by myself and walking up to read my grade. I'd never been as elated as when I saw that "A" for calculus. In many ways, that was a turning point for me. I realized that if I made the effort, did whatever it took, I was going to be able to succeed.

Q: Were people supportive or dismissive?

A: Initially I knew I didn't want to be a surgeon. I liked the variety of being a general practitioner. In the first two years of medical school, you do basic sciences, and you have no contact with patients. I was fortunate that I qualified for a primary care pilot program.

From day one, I was under the lead of a local family physician from Detroit who I met with weekly and had face-to-face contact with. I got to practice my interview skills and clinical skills, and that continued my interest in family medicine. I was fortunate to be in that program with a primary care physician who was great. He introduced me to other local family physicians, so I got contact with patients right off the bat.

I initially went into medical school wanting to be a pediatrician. But, I realized I liked the whole spectrum of patients – not just pediatrics. I wanted to see children and adults.

In family medicine, you can kind of do whatever you want to or whatever your interests are and excel in those. It opens up the ability to take care of the whole patient, versus one spectrum of their health. They may have been more supportive than I knew, but I felt as though it was an uphill battle. I don't think it was a lack of support in the sense of non-support, but I don't think my family knew what I was going to go through and what I did go through. They didn't know how to be more supportive.

My husband was supportive to an extent, but when I decided to do surgery, things started to fall apart. He had told me from the beginning, "You know, if you're going to do surgery, then I won't be able to do this." I ended up going into surgery and we had a hard time for a long time. We eventually divorced during my residency.

Q: What did you enjoy more, the pursuit or the achievement of the activity?

A: By the time the achievement part comes, it's sometimes more about recognition. What I like is the actual work, the actual hard part. I remember when I used to sew clothes when I was little. I'd get the pattern, figure out the material, cut it and sew it, and then by the time I was done it would hang in my closet for a month or two before I wore it. So it wasn't the actual wearing of it I enjoyed, it was the making of it. I do think that's part of my personality.

When I was the president of The American Society for Metabolic and Bariatric Surgery, I worked very, very hard to achieve a new national accreditation program between our society and The American College of Surgeons. I was able to help facilitate a merger of the two. After we had established the joint program and articulated the standards, I stepped back from the committee and the process. I knew that for it to flourish it had to be "owned" by the younger leaders coming up. They had to have a stake in its development.

A year later, my society gave me a big award for quality in surgery. Although it's always wonderful to have your efforts recognized, in essence the award wasn't the point. The fact that patients all over the country and the world can get safe and effective care, that's worth everything. The meaningful part for me was to do it.

This is the theme of my life, pick a hard target/project, and do whatever I need to do to make it happen in the best possible way. Once it's set up and running, I mentor others in how to lead it and step back. In this way, my life is never "done," but there's always growth and progress, and a lifetime of learning. Whatever is around the corner, the next project will be informed by the work on the last one.

Q: Were there ever difficult times in your pursuit?

A: There's nothing quite as difficult as working 110 hours a week as a surgery resident. I remember in my third year of residency, I had two nights off, and it was Christmas and my family needed to see me. I hadn't seen them for a year. I flew home, and I was on edge from being in this intense program, from always working, and from being the only woman in the program.

While I was home, I told my dad, "You know, dad, I think I may not do this. This is a toxic environment, and I'm afraid I might not be able to recover."

He looked at me and said, "Robin, it's painful for you, I know. You're in pain emotionally because you split up with your husband, and physically because you're not getting enough exercise and are working so hard. But remember that if you choose to quit, it'll last a whole lifetime."

That advice got me through that hard moment.

Q: How has being a woman impacted your journey?

A: As a surgery resident, you have to gather all this information so when you go on rounds you know everything about your assigned patients and all your paperwork is done. I'd get up and go in early, because I had to look up all my labs and get all my vital signs. But my male colleagues would come in an hour before their rounds because the nurses would get all that information for them.

There were barriers there, but I was lucky that I had "good hands." In surgery, it's kind of a great equalizer. If you have good hands and a great work effort, you can almost overcome anything, because at the end of the day, if guys know you can operate better than they can, there's a respect that transcends the gender issue.

I believe that in every area of work, there is probably an equalizer. Women just need to find it and then hope that they have an aptitude and put in the hard work to excel.

Now that I've become who I am, I make opportunities for women residents to come and rotate in my clinic, and I try to find good fellowships for women I think would make good teachers and good surgeons. But, they've got to be good candidates; in fact they have to be the best.

I also try to mentor women in all aspects of their careers. My assistant in surgery started with me as an RN and First Assistant, became a Nurse Practitioner and now has her Doctorate of Nursing Practice. In many ways she is just as much a partner in my work as either of my male surgical colleagues. She in turn has become a mentor.

I was the first woman to be president of my surgical society; I was the 26th president. It meant a great deal to me that I'd been voted in by my peers, the vast majority of whom are men.

Q: What's been your greatest accomplishment?

A: The greatest privilege I have is to become a part of the lives of so many people who are in such despair and so sick with their obesity, by performing bariatric surgery. When I'm done, they have such a different path from there on.

The typical person I work with is 150 pounds overweight, has type 2 diabetes, sleep apnea, high blood pressure, and is on multiple medications for coronary artery disease or heart failure. They're often people who have been passed over, even if they're brilliant, for promotions, or their ideas that might be very good aren't taken seriously. It's all because they're big.

They're hurt every day by the reaction of their colleagues and people around them. The cruelty to people who are big is epic. It takes me an hour and a half to do the surgery, and a year later they don't have any of those medical problems anymore.

After the surgery, they fit in.

Q: What was your greatest miscalculation?

A: On a personal level, I missed out on having had children of my own. It's always easy to look back and think, "Wouldn't it be great to have a bunch of kids who are out of college and having their own lives?" But, the truth is, for whatever reason, that wasn't part of the life I was going to have.

Q: What advice would you share with someone who aspired to follow in your footsteps?

A: Consistency of effort and perseverance of effort are important, even when you're not completely sure the goal will be worth it. You have to finish it to know.

Also, you shouldn't spend one minute of your life doing something you're not passionate about. I understand that someone has to take out the garbage, and do the dishes, and it's probably you. But, in terms of the strategy of your life and the day-to-day movement of your life, every day you should do something you believe in.

You have to be passionate about things, and you have to do things you believe in. That unlocks a kind of a secret sauce inside of you. It allows you to unleash some kind of an extraordinary effort or extraordinary talent.

Get in touch with someone you know who has a career in medicine and shadow that person and spend time with him or her on the job. In order to understand what makes medicine different than every other profession, you have to experience the intimacy of the relationship that doctors, nurses, and other health care providers have with their patients. It's that intimacy and relationship that draws you in that makes you accountable and responsible for people.

ACTION GUIDE

An easy reference guide to the advice and tips provided by Dr. Robin Blackstone

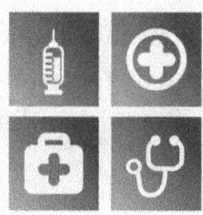

1) Work Through It

Consistency of effort and perseverance of effort are important, even when you're not completely sure the goal will be worth it. You have to finish it to know.

2) Live Everyday Fully

You shouldn't spend one minute of your life doing something you're not passionate about. I understand that someone has to take out the garbage, and do the dishes, and it's probably you. But, in terms of the strategy of your life and the day to day movement of your life, every day you should do something you believe in.

3) Find a Mentor to Shadow

Get in touch with someone you know who has a career in medicine and shadow that person and spend time with him or her on the job.

4) Get Up Close and Personal with Patients

To understand what makes medicine different than every other profession, you have to experience the intimacy of the relationship doctors, nurses, and other health care providers have with their patients.

It's that intimacy and relationship that draws you in that makes you accountable and responsible for people.

5) Read About Others' Experience

There's an eye-opening book by Atul Gawande called *Complications: A Surgeon's Notes on an Imperfect Science*. Another great book, *House of God*, by Samuel Shem, is funny but true. The book called *Forgive and Remember: Managing Medical Failure*, by Charles L. Bosk is also useful.

CHAPTER 2

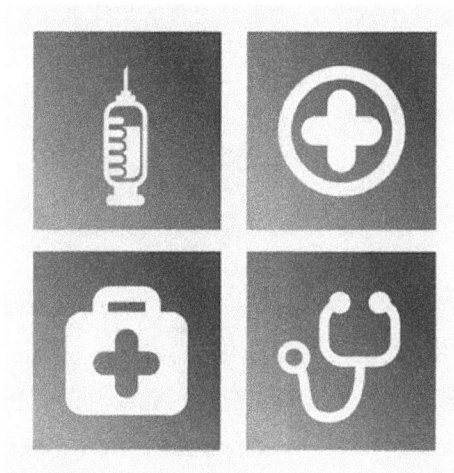

Dr. Robert Cromer

BIOGRAPHY

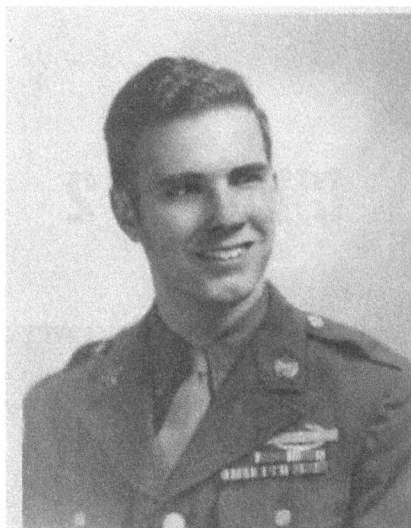

"I decided to be a doctor after the war... I was a combat infantryman in World War II. And, when your friends are killed and you survive, it does something to you. It makes you think to yourself that your life has been spared and you can't waste it. You owe it to your buddies to do something with it the best that you can."

- Dr. Robert Cromer

Dr. Robert Warren Cromer, 1926-2014, was a family physician for 60 years in Antigo, Wisconsin. He is best remembered for his devotion to medicine, his love of nature, his service to his country, and his dedication to balancing his work and family life.

After graduating from high school, Robert enrolled at Northwestern University. Following a year of college, he joined the U.S. Army and served in the 78th Infantry Division during World War II. After sustaining an injury in the Battle of the Bulge, for which he received the Purple Heart, he spent several months in military hospitals, which played a major role in his decision to become a doctor. After his honorable discharge, he returned to Northwestern, where he completed his undergraduate studies and attended medical school. After graduating, he interned at Cook County Hospital in Chicago.

In 1954, Robert moved to Antigo, where he launched his six-decade long family practice. During that time, he delivered more than 3,000 babies and saw tens of thousands of patients. In 1968, he established a clinic at the Antigo Medical Building, and operated it until shortly before his death on June 25, 2014. He was 88 years old.

As an active member of the community, Dr. Cromer was a member of the Langlade County Medical Society and the American Medical Association, and served on the Antigo Unified District School Board. He had a passion for nature and was an avid mountain-climber, hiker, and fisherman. The following interview was conducted just a few weeks before his death.

INTERVIEW

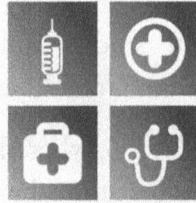

Q: Did you always want to be a doctor?

A: When I was a child, becoming a doctor never entered my mind. I was interested mostly in the outdoors. I became an Eagle Scout, and thought I might become an ornithologist. Then it all changed when World War II began. I was inducted into the Army, went through basic training in Florida, and at age 18, I found myself in the Battle of the Bulge. It was the coldest winter in 100 years, with a foot of snow in the ground. Then, on March 14, 1945, my unit and I were pinned down in a forest by machine gun fire. While I was lying there, a mortar shell came in and a piece of shrapnel hit my leg. I was afraid to look at my leg because I was afraid it was blown off. The guy lying next to me hadn't been hit, so I asked him, "Please take a look. Is my leg still there?"

I can still remember his reply. He said, "You lucky son of a bitch. You got a million dollar wound. "That's a wound that would get you out of the war, but wouldn't cripple you.

During the next several months spent in Army hospitals is when I decided to be a doctor. I still couldn't walk, so I read a lot of detective stories. I thought it was neat to be able to solve these crimes. I thought of how great it would be to solve illnesses, to get the facts, to get the history, to do the examination, and to figure out what the problem was and how to treat it.

Q: Is the war still fresh in your mind?

A: Yes, it's something that never leaves you. I was a combat infantryman, a lowly buck private. When your friends are killed but you survive, it does something to you. It makes you think your life has been spared and you can't waste it. You owe it to your buddies to do the best you can.

Q: What happened when you were released from the hospital?

A: I was fortunate because of my moderate amount of disability that I came under Public Law 16 for education. It paid for my undergraduate education, my medical school education, my books, my supplies, and even a small stipend each month. After that, I graduated from Northwestern.

There was no such thing in those days as a family practice residency. I wanted to be a family practice doctor in a small town. I took a two-year internship at Cook County Hospital. From there, I answered an ad and came up to the Antigo area, where I've been in practice for nearly 60 years.

Q: Why do you enjoy being a doctor?

A: Being a doctor is much more than what I thought it would be. I can't imagine waking up in the morning and not having any reason to get out of bed. There's a certain amount of satisfaction.

The other thing, of course, is that it's what keeps me learning. You should never stop learning. If you do, you become a dinosaur. You've got to keep up, and that helps you feel good about yourself, too

Q: How many patients do you see a day?

A: Nowadays I see no more than five or six a day, but I used to see ten to twenty.

Q: Do you take time in the day for yourself now in between patients?

A: Oh yes, that's when I read medical journals. Everything is changing in medicine today. It's all becoming more esoteric and has to do more with your genes and less with viruses and infections. It's getting more and more technical.

Q: Was passion important in your pursuit of medicine?

A: Yes. Passion is one thing that's important when making the decision to become a doctor. You don't make that decision because you want to do well and help people or because it's a family tradition. Those are okay, but the only thing that's important is that it's something you really want to do; you should be passionate about it.

Q: How much longer do you plan on practicing medicine?

A: That I don't know. It probably won't be a whole lot longer because I don't see a whole lot of patients anymore. I've no plans to quit, but I don't foresee going on a great deal into the future either.

Q: When you started to embark on this path, did you have any doubts?

A: I never had any questions. I was always confident, because I knew I could do whatever I wanted to do.

Q: Where did that confidence come from?

A: I don't think it was something taught to me. One thing that convinced me of that was when I got into mountain climbing. I found that when I climbed mountains I could do more than I ever, ever thought I could. People are capable of many things if they'd just do them.

Q: Were you able to maintain your love of nature as well as practice medicine?

A: Oh yeah, I've done a lot of fishing, hunting, camping and hiking here in Wisconsin. I used to fish in the Wolf River. One year, when my oldest son Steve was a little lad, I took him with me. He was too little to wade and he couldn't fish from the shore. So I put him on my shoulders and carried him out to a raft in the river. Then, finally, when he was tired out, I came out and brought him back to shore.

Many years later my wife and I were visiting our sons. They're both fly fishermen. When I was there, they decided to take me fly fishing up in the mountains on a little river. They packed everything up, got up early in the morning, and took me through some beautiful scenery to get there. I found a place where I could cross the river because it wasn't too deep and there weren't too many rocks.

When it was time to return, I wanted to cross back to the other side, but couldn't find any place. Steve came by and saw what I was doing and said, "Years ago, you took me fishing and you carried me on your back. Now it's my turn." And he carried me piggyback across the river.

Q: Are there lessons you learned in nature that apply to your life and career as well?

A: Yes. I once went hiking on a trail that went around the base of a mountain – about 90 miles long. I hiked part of this trail to an area where I was going to spend the night. I put my sleeping bag out, and I was all alone under the stars. It was great to lie there and see the stars and sky overhead.

I woke up in the morning, and there were a lot of wildflowers growing all over. The birds were singing, the sun was coming up over the mountaintop, and there was a little stream flowing by. I got such a feeling of happiness that it's hard to explain. I felt I should stand there and shout to the whole world how good it was to be alive and where

I was at that time. You can get a similar feeling and satisfaction from the practice of medicine.

Q: If you had to do it over again, would you have done anything differently?

A: I don't think so. Not only do the good things affect your being and your character but the bad things affect you, too. You have to learn how to accept bad things and work around them and accept them as fact. That helps make you who you are.

Q: Is it important for you to do as much as you can in your life?

A: You only go through life once. Take some of the time you have to do the things you dreamed of as a little kid and see the places you want to go. I've been extremely fortunate in my lifetime. I've been able to do more than most people will ever do, and I'm happy being where I am, even though I have health problems now. Nevertheless, I feel good with my life.

Q: What was your greatest failure or miscalculation?

A: I wouldn't trade the good things or the bad things in my life. The bad things have helped make me what I am today, just as well as the good things have. And, I like where I am today. I like myself.

One thing I never counted on – and anybody in medicine is going to come across this eventually because they don't teach much about it – is the heartbreak. Take the woman who delivered a baby and you have to go in and tell her the baby died. Or, you have a young family whose four-year-old son is their pride and joy in their life, and you have to tell them that, although he only got sick yesterday, he died of meningococcal meningitis.

Those are the things I never counted on and that aren't taught in school. But, as a doctor, you have to do them because that's part of your duty. You have to relay the bad news. You can't put that off on somebody else; that's part of being a doctor.

Q: Is there anything else medical school didn't prepare you for?

A: One of the things you don't learn in medical school is the art of medicine. The technology and everything you learn, that's the body of medicine – your classes and your knowledge. The art of medicine is the soul of medicine. It's getting to know your patients, treating them right, and knowing each one as an individual.

For those going to medical school today, by the time they graduate there's so much debt that they don't have as much time as we did in my day. The doctors of today can't afford to spend time with their patients because they're so deeply in debt. They have to see too many patients per day.

Q: What was your greatest success or accomplishment?

A: Not any one thing. It's all together. It's all about my patients. For instance, many years ago, I delivered a baby who was premature. She only weighed about a pound. We didn't have intensive care nurseries then, but we had a regular nursery. I'd taken care of her and the nurses did. That was what saved her.

About fifteen years later, my wife and I were eating in a restaurant when this pretty young girl came up to the table and said, "My parents said I should come over here and introduce myself." She was that premature girl.

It blows my mind. Another time, a man came up to me in public and said, "You're my hero." That blew me away. He was a patient of mine. I've seen people where I've treated their mother and their grandmother, and in some instances maybe even their great grandmother over time. I've delivered more than 3,000 babies.

It's things like that where I feel, at least to some extent, that my life has mattered. That's my accomplishment. I haven't gotten any big awards like others have. But, my awards are what my patients have said and done, and through letters they've written to me.

Q: What advice would you give to those who want to follow in your footsteps?

A: One of the most important things is to make a pact with yourself that you're willing to take the time and the effort to get to your goal and then to continue on. When I think about time, no matter how much of it you put into medicine, you've got to take time alone and away to smell the roses and run barefoot through the fields of gold.

Never let medicine get between you and your family. What's important is to find time if you have a family, even if you're busy. Somehow I was able to spend a lot of time with my family. Those things come back to you years later.

I remember one medical school class reunion where they had asked all the doctors to write down the most important thing in their lives. Many were famous, but the majority of them wrote that the most important thing in their life was family, believe it or not.

Take time to read to your kids. You can always find a little time. My youngest son, John, was in third grade when I read him *The Hobbit*. I'd come home every evening or late afternoon and, as soon as I'd come through the door, I'd get the book and we'd sit on the couch and I'd read the next chapter. He later read *The Lord of the Rings* and got me to read it. I can't encourage people enough to read, if nothing else.

Q: Is there anything in particular you'd recommend future doctors read?

A: Read about the life of Albert Schweitzer. He became a doctor later in life. He was a concert organist and was also a clergyman. He decided to quit his job and become a doctor. Then he went to Africa and set up a little hospital and spent the rest of his life there. He was awarded the Nobel Peace Prize and he used the money awarded to add on to his hospital there. Knowing that medicine produces people like that and you're a part of a heritage is important.

When you finish medical school, you're standing on top of a pyramid. And that pyramid was built by all the people who came before you. One day you'll be one of the predecessors and someone else will be standing higher on the pyramid. All of that is to help you understand where you are, where you're coming from, and where you're going.

ACTION GUIDE

An easy reference guide to the advice and tips provided by Dr. Robert Cromer

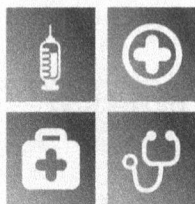

1) Make a Pact with Yourself to Succeed

One of the most important things is to make a pact with yourself that you're willing to take the time and the effort to get to your goal and then to continue on. When I think about time, no matter how much of it you put into medicine, you've got to take time alone and away to smell the roses and run barefoot through the fields of gold.

2) Put Family First

Never let medicine get between you and your family. What's important is to find time if you have a family, even if you're busy. Somehow I was able to spend a lot of time with my family. Those things come back to you years later.

3) Take Time to Read to Your Kids

You can always find a little time. My youngest son, John, was in third grade when I read him *The Hobbit*. I'd come home every evening or late afternoon, and as soon as I'd got in I'd get the book and we'd sit on the couch and I'd read the next chapter. He later read *The Lord of the Rings* and got me to read it. I can't encourage people enough to read, if nothing else.

4) Be an Example

When you finish medical school, you're standing on top of a pyramid. And that pyramid was built by all the people who came before you. One day you'll be one of the predecessors and somebody else will be standing higher on the pyramid. All of that is to help you understand where you are, where you're coming from, and where you're going.

5) Prepare for the Heartbreak

One thing I never counted on – and anybody in medicine is going to come across this eventually because they don't teach much about it – is the heartbreak. You have to relay the bad news. You can't put that off on somebody else; that's part of being a doctor.

CHAPTER 3

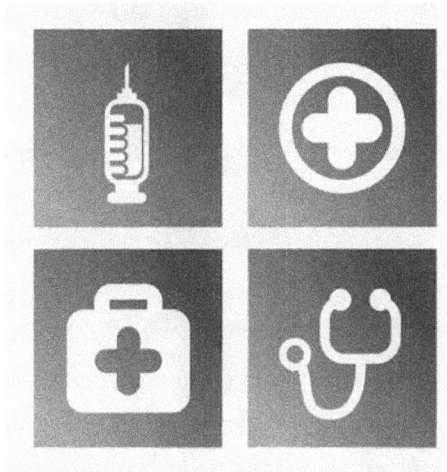

Dr. Matthew Hummel

BIOGRAPHY

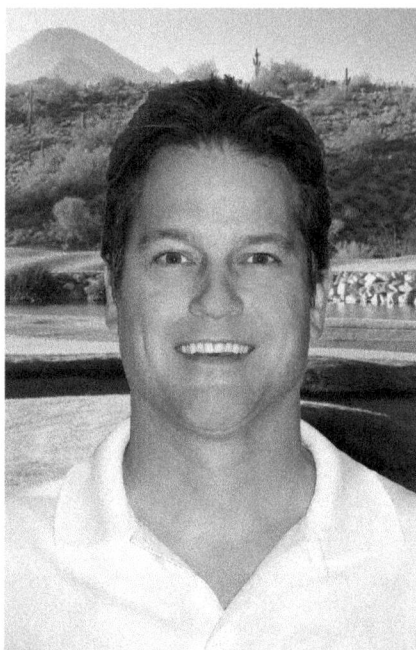

"Believe in yourself. There's always going to be somebody smarter, there's always going to be somebody who gets a better grade, and there's always going to be somebody out there who could intimidate you if you allow it. You have to have confidence in yourself that you can be the best physician that you can be."

- Dr. Matthew Hummel

Matthew Hummel is an allopathic physician in Fountain Hills, Arizona, specializing in family medicine. He is also the Principal Investigator for Synexus, a medical research company, and the Medical Director of Savior Hospice Care.

Dr. Hummel received his Bachelor of Science degree in physiology from Michigan State University. He then went to Wayne State University School of Medicine. He completed his residency at St.

Joseph's Hospital in Phoenix, then went to work as an M.D. with Scottsdale Healthcare in a family practice.

In 2002, after only three years as a physician, Dr. Hummel established the Fountain Hills Family Practice P.C., a full-service primary care medical operation, which had a staff of 32 people and more than 15,000 patients.

Dr. Hummel has been featured in *Phoenix Magazine* as a 'Top Doctor' on ten occasions. As recently as 2017, he was voted the top family doctor. He has also been featured in *Scottsdale 101* magazine as the 'Number Two Family Physician' in the entire Phoenix area. In 2010, Dr. Hummel was the Preceptor of the Year for Arizona State University.

In 2017, Dr. Hummel decided to change his practice to a concierge practice, joining MDVIP in June of that year. He now has 600 patients in his practice.

INTERVIEW

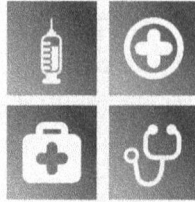

Q: How long have you been practicing family medicine?

A: I received my medical degree in 1996, finished my residency in 1999, so I've been practicing on my own for more than 19 years.

Q: What is your staff comprised of?

A: I currently have four employees: a front office/office manager, a biller/medical assistant, another medical assistant, and a registered nurse. My wife, Suzanne, handles the business side of the practice.

Q: What was behind your decision to switch to a concierge practice?

A: First of all, it allows me to spend more time with each patient and to also have more time for my family. I see patients the same day or, for urgent matters, the next day. This new model of medicine allows for longer office visits for each patient and gives me time to address each patient's medical, physical and psychological concerns.

I also do an annual complete physical exam through Cleveland Clinic Heart Clinic, which includes advanced testing in my office, along with advanced lab work. I can now be much more proactive with my patients' health, and spend significantly more time with my patients, providing the preventive care they deserve.

Q: Did you get any training in medical school on being self-employed?

A: You don't get any training on that. It's trial and error. It's about knowing people, knowing personalities, and working with those personalities.

I'm in a field where patients need to have a pleasant experience – they already don't feel well. It's an important thing, from the front desk all the way to the check-out. The patients have to be treated with respect and kindness. Patients are often focused on their ailments, but my employees understand that the patients don't feel well so they're able to be more empathetic to their situation.

Q: Would it be difficult for you to go back and work for someone else?

A: I'd never do it unless I was at the end of my career and I wanted to slow down. It would have to be the right time and the right financial incentive. But, I have no desire to work for anybody at this time.

Q: Will you please describe your typical day?

A: My day starts at 8 a.m. Monday through Thursday. I see patients every 30 minutes or, in the case of an annual exam, 90 minutes. I take 12 noon to 1 p.m. for lunch, meetings and patient call-backs. I then do the same schedule from 1 to 5 p.m. I typically see 10 to 12 patients a day. This is much better than the 25-30 patients a day my traditional practice demanded. September through June, we have a half day on Friday, while we're closed Fridays during July and August.

Q: How did you get started on your career path?

A: I became interested in medicine in general in the first part of high school, and I enjoyed sciences and did well in them. I also had good mentors as teachers. My next-door neighbor was a surgeon I was very fond of, and I was interested in his career.

After I finished high school, I attended Michigan State University and obtained a Bachelor of Science in physiology. I then went to Wayne State University School of Medicine in Detroit. After completing four years of medical school, I did a residency at St. Joseph's Hospital in Phoenix, Arizona. When I finished my residency, I took a job with Scottsdale Healthcare in Fountain Hills, Arizona.

Q: What sparked your interest in science?

A: In ninth grade, I took an anatomy and physiology class with a great teacher, Dr. Rathbun. I learned about the anatomy, physiology, and function of the human body. It was fascinating. I then had a physics and chemistry professor, Mr. Hopkins, who was great.

In tenth grade, I'd also volunteer and follow Dr. Wolf, my neighbor, who was a general surgeon. I'd follow him around at the hospital and kind of see what he did. At that time in school, I was doing well and had my eye on becoming a doctor.

Q: Did you always know you wanted to be a general practitioner?

A: Initially I knew I didn't want to be a surgeon. I liked the variety of being a general practitioner. In the first two years of medical school, you do basic sciences, and you have no contact with patients. I was fortunate that I qualified for a primary care pilot program.

From day one, I was under the lead of a local family physician from Detroit who I met with weekly and had face-to-face contact with. I got to practice my interview skills and clinical skills, and that continued my interest in family medicine. I was fortunate to be in that program with a primary care physician who was great. He introduced me to other local family physicians, so I got contact with patients right off the bat.

I initially went into medical school wanting to be a pediatrician. But, I realized I liked the whole spectrum of patients – not just pediatrics. I wanted to see children and adults.

In family medicine, you can kind of do whatever you want to or whatever your interests are and excel in those. It opens up the ability to take care of the whole patient, versus one spectrum of their health.

Q: Was passion important in the pursuit of your goals?

A: I definitely had a passion for it. Both undergraduate school and medical school are grueling, and the volume of work is massive. So, you have to have a passion for what you're doing. If you don't, you'll never be happy.

Unfortunately, I do see physicians who aren't happy in their pursuit. Passion isn't there, wasn't there, or weakened over time. But, I still love going to work every day. I look forward to it, and I enjoy it. As long as that passion continues to be there, I plan on working.

At the end of the day, the most important thing if you do go into medicine is that you go into it knowing it will be a long road. Know that you have to do it, not because your mom and dad want you to, or you feel it's something you have to, but because you want to do it.

Also, make sure you don't look at the financial aspects of the different specialties, but find something you have passion for. It doesn't matter how much money you make if you're doing something every day you don't enjoy. It'll get old. If people have the passion, the desire, the ability, and follow their passions for the right reasons, they'll be successful and will enjoy what they do.

Q: Were you apprehensive about becoming a doctor?

A: No one in my family had ever been a doctor, so I was a little unsure of what to do and who to talk to. It was trial by fire, initially. But, having those three folks who were so influential in my learning helped push me toward it. Plus, my parents were supportive in whatever I wanted to do. It was nice that when I picked something I was interested in they were always supportive.

Q: Did you ever want to give up?

A: No one in my family had ever been a doctor, so I was a little unsure of what to do and who to talk to. It was trial by fire, initially. But, having those three folks who were so influential in my learning helped push me toward it. Plus, my parents were supportive in whatever I wanted to do. It was nice that when I picked something I was interested in they were always supportive.

There were always moments where I did poorly on a test. I went from being "top dog" in high school and college to medical school, where everybody was the "top dog" in their schools. It took a while for me to realize I wasn't competing with my peers but with myself.

Once I realized that, I became much more involved with my career, as opposed to being constantly intimidated by someone who would do better on a test or someone who was smarter. That was the hardest thing in the beginning of medical school. Once I realized that, that competition, that fear, and that apprehension went out the window.

Q: If you had to do it all again, what would you do differently?

A: I'd have spent more time during residency learning different procedures. I would have liked to have the opportunity to travel to Central America where other doctors go and serve the under-privileged of the world. But, I couldn't pick a better place to be, or have a more successful practice. I'm fortunate that way.

Q: What's been one of your greatest successes or accomplishments?

A: I've been fortunate to be successful in a great small town, and I've gathered a following and have been known as the doctor to go to in Fountain Hills. This allowed me to transition to a concierge practice. I have good patient feedback and a great staff that makes medicine enjoyable again. I'm most proud of how I've built my practice to the level it is now.

Q: What's been your greatest miscalculation?

A: My greatest miscalculation would have to be the lack of business studies or business academic exposure I have. Unfortunately, medicine is a business. So, learning the business of medicine is somewhat foreign in most divisions and was probably the most difficult.

Fortunately, I've learned to hire good people and who I can get information from when I don't know it. I've been lucky with the people who have helped me along the way: accountants, attorneys, office managers, and business managers. They have helped in areas where I was lacking. If you can't do the business of medicine, you can't pay the bills, and you can't practice medicine. So, they go hand in hand.

Most doctors get out of residency wanting to be employed by someone, so they have the comfort of a paycheck and 401K, and no worries beyond just seeing patients. A lot of people are comfortable with that. But I find that if you can master both aspects, it becomes much more rewarding – both personally and financially. It allows you to enjoy the practice of medicine.

Q: What advice would you give to those who aspire to follow in your footsteps?

A: Number one, have a mentor, or somebody you look up to, who has a passion for what he or she does and has been successful. A mentor can also tell you the good and the bad, to a degree.

Also, believe in yourself. There's always going to be someone smarter, someone who gets a better grade, and someone who could intimidate you if you allow it. You have to have that complete confidence in yourself that you can be the best physician possible.

In medical school there's a ton of information. No one can learn it all. Learn how to study and gather information as a whole, as opposed to concerning yourself with the exact specifics of everything. That will allow you to gather information you can home in on over time.

I find that in the practice of medicine there's a big difference between knowing the book and knowing how to be a physician. You need to know the information, obviously, and you need to be well-read with diagnoses and treatment. But, you also have to have the personality and the ability to gather information from patients so they feel comfortable in uncomfortable medical situations, so you can get the correct information and formulate an assessment and plan.

If you can do that with patients and they feel comfortable with you, they'll be compliant with your treatment. That's a lot better. That's when it becomes fun – when patients come in not feeling well, then leave feeling a bit better, and over time, with the correct diagnoses and treatment, they succeed. That's when it's all worth it. And, that's with life in general.

At the end, it doesn't always happen. It's realizing that if you do the best you can, you'll have good outcomes. You'll have to deal with bad outcomes when they occur, but not dwelling on that is important as well.

Q: What resources would you suggest for someone who wants a career in medicine?

A: If you have an interest in medicine, go to your local hospital. Volunteer in different aspects of medicine to see what interests you. When I was a volunteer in high school, I did rotations in neurology, emergency medicine, general surgery, and in many other things. I realized pretty quickly that I didn't want to be a neurologist and I didn't want to be an ER doctor.

Getting exposure will help you decide. It's important to not be dead-set on one specific area of medicine until you get a feel for that specialty, because you may find it's not what you expected.

Also, talk to people in the field. Talk to other doctors and teachers who have a passion for what they do. Finding a good mentor is primary to being successful in any career you pick.

Q: What do you think of telemedicine?

A: It's an interesting idea. With the limited time we're able to spend with patients these days, having the ability to have some form of live feed for a physician would be an excellent idea. But, the inability to touch and examine the patient would be somewhat difficult to do without the physical presence of the patient.

A lot of medicine and diagnosis is based on patients' history and the questions they answer – the positives and the negatives. Telemedicine negates the need, in a lot of cases, for a physical exam per se. I can see it being helpful. It could be a great option for patients who are willing to consider that type of medicine.

ACTION GUIDE

An easy reference guide to the advice and tips provided by Dr. Matthew Hummel

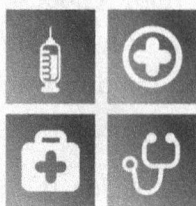

1) Have a Mentor

Have a mentor or someone you look up to who has a passion for what he or she does and has been successful. A mentor can also tell you the good and the bad, to a degree.

2) Learn How to Study

In medical school, there is a ton of information. No one can learn it all. Learn how to study and gather information as a whole, as opposed to concerning yourself with the exact specifics of everything. That will allow you to gather information you can home in on over time.

3) Expand Your Medical Knowledge Base

Spend more time during residency learning different procedures. I would have liked to have the opportunity to travel to Central America where other doctors go and get to serve the under-privileged of the world.

4) Expand Your Business Knowledge

Spend more time in school learning business skills. My greatest miscalculation would have to be the lack of business studies or business academic exposure I have. Unfortunately, medicine is a business. So, learning the business of medicine is somewhat foreign in most divisions and was probably the most difficult.

5) Believe in Yourself

Believe in yourself. There's always going to be someone smarter, someone who gets a better grade, and someone who could intimidate you if you allow it. You have to have that complete confidence in yourself that you can be the best physician possible.

CHAPTER 4

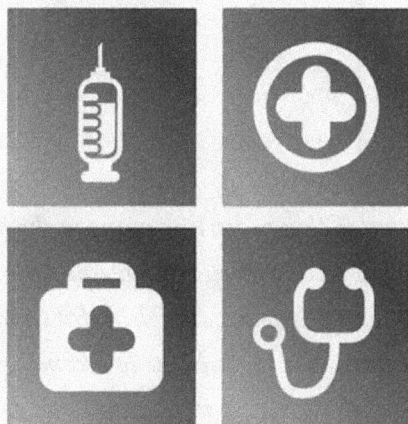

Jessie Koljonen

BIOGRAPHY

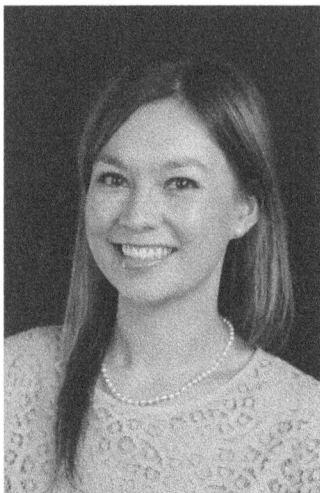

"I also learned that if things don't go my way the first time, to not give up right away. I have to keep trying, especially if I'm passionate about what I'm doing. It was valuable; I did stumble and fail at first, but I learned the ingredients to becoming successful."

– Jessie Koljonen

Jessie Koljonen is a third-year medical student at the University of Arizona College of Medicine – Phoenix. She is a candidate for the Certificate of Distinction in Service and Community Health, working with the underserved population and learning how to overcome barriers to care. She also served as the interest group leader for several medical specialty groups, and helped organize teen pregnancy classes at the county hospital. She is currently doing her clinical rotations and is undecided what specialty she would like to pursue.

Koljonen graduated from college with a double major in Behavioral Biology and Spanish from Johns Hopkins University in Baltimore, Maryland. After college, she pursued a Master's Degree in Biomedical

Sciences from Tufts University in Boston, Mass. She worked at MeMD as the Clinical and Service Operations Manager, where she handled routine follow-up patient calls and clinical quality.

Prior to attending university, Koljonen studied at the Peggy Payne Academy, a highly selective high school, and interned at a neuroscience lab at Arizona State University.

In 2011, she became the District 6 winner of the City of Phoenix Outstanding Young Woman of the Year. While at Johns Hopkins, she interned in the Admissions Office, served as VP of Committees in Phi Mu, was a member of the Blue Key Society, acted as an admissions representative, was an Alumni Student Ambassador, a Research Assistant in a Neuroscience Lab at the Medical Campus, and worked at the Children's House at the JHU children's hospital.

INTERVIEW

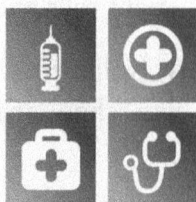

Q: How would you describe your typical day?

A: I don't have a typical day. Right now I'm working on compliance at MeMD, a leading telemedicine company which allows patients to see a doctor online or over the phone. I'm currently developing policies and procedures for privacy, security, and recertification that are required by HIPAA, HITECH, and the Omnibus Rule. I'm also implementing staff training to make sure everyone understands HIPAA and to make sure we're compliant with all the states where we provide services.

I also do patient follow-up calls every week to make sure everything is okay, that they filled their prescriptions, don't have any side effects, and to make sure there's no need for further follow up. So, I do enjoy that chance for patient interaction, which is what I crave in wanting to be a doctor.

I also oversee clinical quality, where I ensure our providers are abiding by our prescription policies. Telemedicine is a little different than practicing in a clinic or hospital, and it's such a new field that it requires a lot of educating for both patients and providers, so I want to make sure we're following the standards and guidelines we've set. As far as the rest of my job description- it's a team effort here at MeMD; so for any project that needs my help, I hop on board.

Q: When did you know you wanted to be a doctor?

A: When I was in high school, I was able to work at the neuroscience lab at ASU, and that was what sparked my interest in neuroscience and in neurosurgery as well. My first day in the lab was cool. I walked in and saw they were doing emergency brain dissections on all these rats.

I walked in with my guidance counselor and she was so grossed out, and I thought I'd be, too, but when I walked in I was so amazed and energized. I thought for a second, "Hmm, this might be something I'd be interested in doing."

From there, I went to Johns Hopkins University in Baltimore, where I started to pursue a major in neuroscience. Hopkins has a great neuroscience program, so it took off from there.

Q: What type of neurosurgeon do you want to be?

A: The thing about neurosurgery is that even though it's a quite specific field, it can get even more specific. The neurosurgeon I shadowed was a cerebral-vascular neurosurgeon. Basically, her most typical procedure was clipping aneurisms. That's one type of neurosurgery, and I'm sure I probably don't even know about all the different types. That's what medical school is for – to try all those things out to make sure that's what I want to do.

Q: I like your perspective on that. Students should feel free to explore as much as possible in medical school. How are your plans working out so far?

A: When I visualized my career path, I thought I'd go to Hopkins, graduate, get a 4.0 in neuroscience, with maybe some other majors thrown in there, go to med school right away, and become a superstar surgeon. Obviously, I haven't done all of it yet, but I visualized a straightforward path. You know, it hasn't always worked out that way, but I think the bumps in the road enriched my journey.

Q: What were some of the 'bumps in the road'?

A: When I got to Hopkins I was 'gung-ho' about being a neuroscience major and a career as a brain surgeon. My first year at Hopkins threw me for a loop. The classes were a lot harder than I had expected. I didn't do well. It opened my eyes again about how it's not a straight path and won't be as easy as I thought it was going to be.

After my freshman year, I had to do some soul searching and I thought, "Was neuroscience what I wanted to do? Do I want to be involved in medicine? Do I want to be a doctor? Do I want to be a surgeon? Can I do it? Clearly, it's not working out for me at Hopkins." Definitely, after my first year, I had major doubts and you could say this was a hiccup in my plan.

Q: How did you overcome it?

A: After my first year, I switched majors and I sought advice from a few people. It's nice having some support. I spoke to my parents, who were supportive of whatever I chose, and then I met with a few trusted professors at Hopkins.

One of them was the chair of the Neuroscience and Behavioral Biology program, and Behavioral Biology is what I ended up majoring in. She was enthusiastic and excited about neuroscience. Being able to talk to someone like that also got me excited about my topic. She opened my eyes to behavioral biology – not totally putting away neuroscience but broadening my horizons a little bit.

The second thing I did was to reach out to a neurosurgeon at the Hopkins hospital. I'd been lucky to be able to shadow her basically my entire time at Hopkins University. That was probably the best experience in terms of the career path I've been on, in terms of advice, and in terms of the mentoring she's given me.

I talked to her about how she became a neurosurgeon, the bumps in the road she experienced, and how she got to where she is today. She was probably the biggest influence in terms of who I talked to and who gave me the best advice.

After I graduated, she encouraged me to continue our communication; she'd already been through what I was experiencing at that point, and wanted to help out in any way she could. It's cool to be able to have that resource available.

Q: Is passion important in the pursuit of a career?

A: It's important, especially if you're spending so many hours dedicated to studying. Passion definitely needs to play a key part in what you're doing. In terms of any job, you want to be passionate or at least interested in what you're doing or you'll be bored to tears.

My mentor, the neurosurgeon I've been able to shadow, gave me a piece of advice one day. She told me, "Jessie, I'm not a morning person. I hate getting up. It's hard for me to get out of bed early in the morning, but I found a job that I love so much it makes me excited to get up, to go to work, to operate on people."

I thought about that. She was obviously saying she's doing something she's passionate about. That struck a chord with me. I never used to be a morning person, but now I am. I want to find a job like that, or I want to be a surgeon and want to wake up in the morning and be excited about treating patients and saving lives.

Q: What has been your greatest accomplishment to this point?

A: My greatest success thus far was graduating from Hopkins. It was long and difficult, but it was worth it. Other than that, my other accomplishment was being able to shadow a neurosurgeon throughout my time in college. It was cool because I was able to see the different aspects of what she did.

I thought that all surgeons did was operate every day. They go into the OR, they leave and go home, and then come back and do more surgeries. But I learned they also attend conferences with other neurosurgeons, and they talk about all these cool technologies and upcoming techniques they're working on.

I shadowed my mentor and attended pre-op rounds and post-op rounds, where she'd go and see patients before and after operations. She also had clinics where she saw patients, reviewed their charts, recommended what their next course of treatment would be, and things like that. I got to see all different aspects of what she did.

Q: What were some things that happened along the way that you couldn't have predicted but proved to be valuable in their pursuit?

A: I thought I came from a quite gifted high school program. I got pretty decent grades to get into Hopkins. So, I thought it would be pretty much the same: I'd study a little bit and I'd be able to do the same things I was doing. Then when I got to Hopkins, I realized it was a totally different atmosphere.

I wasn't prepared to take on the academic course load Hopkins offered. I had to totally revamp my studying skills and habits. Before, when I studied, I'd read the textbook chapter the night before an exam, review my notes, take the test, and I'd be fine with it. At Hopkins, though, I had to learn to understand the material and not just regurgitate the information, and how to understand the concepts and how they apply to other concepts. That's a skill that will help me wherever I go.

I also learned that if things don't go my way the first time, to not give up right away. I have to keep trying, especially if I'm passionate about what I'm doing. It was valuable; I did stumble and fail at first, but I learned the ingredients to becoming successful.

Q: If you had to do it again, would you do anything differently?

A: I wouldn't do anything differently, because even the things I thought I wanted to do differently I learned from. In the end, everything happens for a reason. The first year, when I didn't do well academically at Hopkins, I wouldn't have changed that, because it might not have made me so passionate to pursue shadowing a surgeon or to pursue a different major and the different classes I ended up choosing.

Q: Do you have any advice for aspiring physicians?

A: The first piece of advice is to find a mentor in your desired specialty, because a mentor has been through the same thing you're going through and could probably give you some insight nobody else could. A mentor also helps put things in perspective and reminds you of that light at the end of the tunnel – your long term goal.

A second piece of advice, following up with the mentoring thing, would be to ask questions and be informed. I started out wanting to study neuroscience and I wasn't sure. But, if you ask questions, that's how you choose your major, and it's how you develop that passion you have. At least that's how I did it.

My third piece of advice is a big one. If it doesn't happen right away like you'd expect it to, don't give up – especially if you believe it's what you want to do. Most things in life that are worth it aren't easy. It's worth the struggle to find the end of the tunnel. Plus, everything happens for a reason. So, don't give up right away. If it's meant to be, it'll happen. You have to work a little bit harder.

The other thing would be to know your strengths. I know I'm a hard worker, for example, but I know I'm not the smartest person in the room. So, I know I have to work extra hard in order to get the grades I want. If you know your strengths, and your weaknesses, it can help you adapt to your culture and your classes, or to whatever you're pursuing. That can help you be successful.

Q: What resources would you recommend for aspiring physicians?

A: The best resource is finding someone who's currently in the position you're looking to pursue. That's where you'll get the first-hand advice. Certain blogs or other resources might not portray the inevitable hardships you'll encounter as a medical student; they're mostly designed to draw students into medicine and might only show you the positives. But, people who've been through it will tell you the struggles they've had to get to where they are.

Having a support group, especially with someone who's going through the same thing you're going through, is important. I'm currently studying for the MCAT. I'm retaking it. I have a friend who retook it as well. So, we've been motivating each other.

It helps to have others you can relate to. If you don't score so well on a practice exam, you can reach out to them. Or, if you scored well, they can cheer you on, too. Having a peer in the same boat as you is also helpful.

ACTION GUIDE

An easy reference guide to the advice and tips provided by Dr. Jessie Koljonen

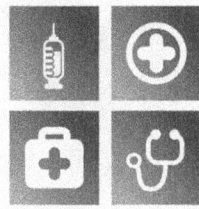

1) Find a Mentor

Find a mentor, because a mentor has been through the same thing you're going through and can probably give you some insight nobody else can.

2) Ask Questions

Ask questions and be informed. If you ask questions, that's how you change your major, and it's how you develop that passion you have.

3) Know Your Strengths

You may have to work extra hard to get the grades you want. If you know your strengths, and your weaknesses, it can help you adapt to your culture and your classes, or to whatever you're pursuing. That can help you be successful.

4) Have a Support Group

Having a support group, especially with someone who's going through the same thing you're going through at the same time, is important. Having a peer in the same boat as you is usually very helpful.

5) Don't Give Up

Don't give up – especially if you believe it's what you want to do. Most things in life that are worth it aren't easy. It's worth the struggle to find the end of the tunnel. Plus, everything happens for a reason. So, don't give up right away. If it's meant to be, it'll happen. You have to work a little bit harder.

CHAPTER 5

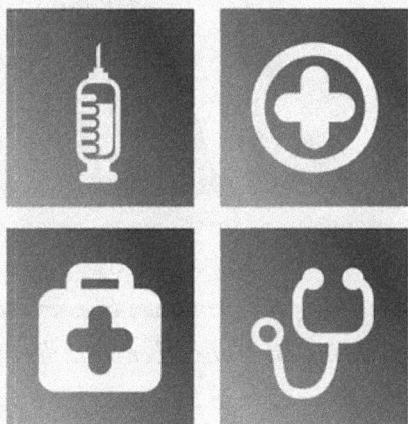

Dr. Rachel Lindor

BIOGRAPHY

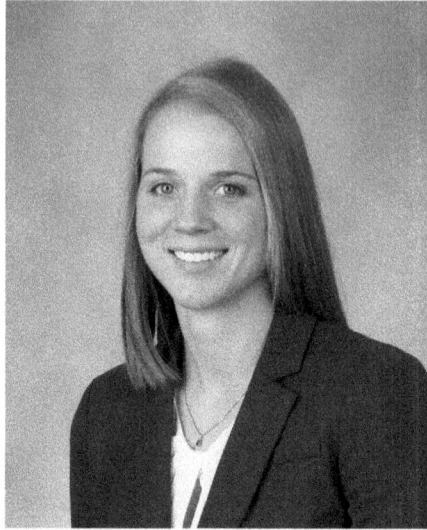

"If you're doing something you genuinely like, are curious about, and gives you energy, then a lot of the other obstacles fall away. If you fail at something, do terribly in a class, or get a paper rejected, it doesn't matter, because you're just doing it because you're interested in it and it drives you. It's really important because it allows you to overcome a lot of the hurdles you hit along the way."

– Dr. Rachel Lindor

Dr. Rachel Lindor holds degrees in both law and medicine. She recently completed a residency in emergency medicine at the famed Mayo Clinic in Rochester, Minnesota and currently works as an emergency medicine physician at the Mayo Clinic in Phoenix, Arizona. She looks forward to combining her clinical and legal backgrounds for a career in health policy.

Dr. Lindor grew up in Rochester. Both her parents were physicians, and she knew she'd have a future in medicine. However, her career path to medicine was not a straight line. She attended the College of Saint Benedict/Saint John's University. While an English major, she was immersed in the sciences and was in the pre-medicine program.

Early on in college, she read Tracy Kidder's *Mountains Beyond Mountains,* a book tracing the life of a physician and anthropologist focused on providing healthcare to indigent populations abroad. Thinking these books exaggerated the extent of health disparities abroad, she spent her summers in college in rural Uganda and Thailand to see for herself. Her experiences there reinforced her desire to make a difference through health policy. From that point forward, she read every book she could get her hands on about international and domestic health policies.

Lindor attended the Mayo Medical School after completing her undergraduate degree. During that time, she spent much of her free time working with uninsured patients and eventually started a free clinic that has since been incorporated into the medical students' curriculum to improve patients' access to care and to increase medical students' exposure to underserved populations and the problems they face.

Two years into medical school, she chose to pursue a law degree as a complement to her medical training, and matriculated into the Sandra Day O'Connor College of Law at Arizona State University, graduating with a Juris Doctorate in 2011, ranked second in her class, and recognized as the "Top Law Student" by the university. She also received the Daniel Strouse Prize at graduation, an award by the law school's Center for Law, Science & Innovation. The $10,000 award is annually made to the student whose academic strengths, contributions to the center and personal qualities most closely mirror those of Strouse, a longtime center director and professor who died of cancer.

Following graduation, Dr. Lindor spent nine months using her law degree in Washington, D.C, working in the Immediate Office of the Secretary for the Department of Health and Human Services, where she devised innovative reimbursement policies for new medical devices. She then spent another nine months working at the law school at Arizona State University, serving as the Research Director for the Center for Law, Science, and Innovation, and teaching law students in the "Genetics and Law" course. She remains affiliated with the law school as a research fellow.

Lindor returned to the Mayo Clinic in 2013 to complete her medical training, graduating from medical school in 2014 and from residency in 2017. During her training, she authored more than 25 peer-review articles, was named the Teacher of the Quarter multiple times, and was recognized nationally as the Best Resident Researcher by the Society for Academic Emergency Medicine.

INTERVIEW

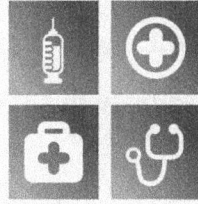

Q: Where are you on your career path?

A: Right now, I'm working as an emergency room physician at the Mayo Clinic in Phoenix, Arizona, but I'd like to eventually do something that combines my clinical background with my legal background. It may be some type of career in health policy – whether that's working with the government part time or just working for a hospital and trying to improve the regulatory and legal structures our health care systems give us. Because I change my mind a lot, I just call it "vague ambition in health policy."

Q: When did you decide to pursue policy and health?

A: It wasn't until pretty late that I decided to pursue policy and health. I grew up in Rochester, Minnesota, which is dominated by Mayo and I had parents who worked with Mayo. At an early age I thought, "Oh, I'll do medicine." So, that was my default. I like medicine, I like working with people, and I like science. It was a good fit.

Then, in college, I read a book written by a doctor who worked in developing countries, and he poignantly described the disparities in healthcare and the quality of life that exists in these countries. Until that point, I'd been pretty sheltered.

Reading that book was eye-opening for me, and I almost didn't believe it because I was used to Rochester and running the halls of Mayo. I couldn't believe what he was describing could be true. I thought the book was an exaggeration. That's why I had to see it for myself.

Q: What did you see and how did it impact you?

A: Over the next couple of summers, I lived for a few weeks in different developing countries. It was those trips abroad and living in rural countryside Uganda when I realized this was not an exaggeration; these people have no resources. If they get sick, there's no healthcare there. It seemed overwhelming.

I ended up being interested in international health care. I read every book I could get my hands on about international health policies – hundreds of them. Reading that pushed me more toward thinking about domestic issues and access to health care and disparity here.

I thought, "If I want to make a difference in this arena, I should be a macroeconomist and work on the country's trade regulations; or, I could be a civil engineer and work on their water supply." But, those aren't the things I'm interested in. I love the policy stuff, and I like medical care. If I'd decided to be a macroeconomist – which I'd hate – maybe I'd be able to do it, but probably not that well. But, at the end of the day, you have to follow what you enjoy.

So, I decided I still want to pursue medicine, but I was also interested in the medical delivery system, and I was trying to figure out how to remedy these disparities in healthcare and access to healthcare.

Q: Were you apprehensive about pursuing both medicine and law?

A: No I wasn't at first. I was too young. I wasn't sure what I was getting myself into. Anyone who knows me will say I'm incredibly stubborn. I was interested in it and wanted to do it, so I made up my mind. I'd say I was confident I was going to do it.

Mayo, where I started medical school, was good about letting you transfer after your second year and get any other degree you thought would be helpful or interesting. I chose to do a law degree. Then I took another year off to work and use it.

Q: Was law school different than medical school?

A: In medical school, I found everyone was following the leader. They were doing what they should be doing and had this mentality of "keep your head down and get your work done." But in law school, there were so many people who were clearly passionate about random things and were doing amazing stuff. Experiencing this difference between medical school and law school, and being in that environment, was helpful for me.

It was the first time I'd been around people like that who were doing their own thing because they were interested in it and had no other driving force.

Q: What did you do when you were working with the government?

A: For a while, I worked for the Department of Health and Human Services (HHS). I was working behind some political appointees, and I ended up being an extension of them in the immediate office of the HHS Secretary. It was tied to Obama's Small Business Initiative and the goal was to come up with innovative reimbursement policies for new medical devices.

It sounds super-boring to most people, but I loved it. It was fascinating and I had a hard time leaving. I ended up working with them for nine months, and then remotely for another two years on that specific policy.

Q: How much of a role does passion play in what you do?

A: I tend to avoid the word "passion," because I think it's overused. But as far as having strong interest in law and medicine, yes I do! If you're doing something you genuinely like, are curious about, and it gives you energy, then a lot of the obstacles fall away. Being told you're not doing something right doesn't matter if you're doing what you're interested in.

If you fail at something, do terribly in a class, or get a paper rejected, it doesn't matter. You're doing it because you're interested in it and it drives you. It allows you to overcome a lot of the hurdles you hit along the way.

Q: How did people react when they learned you were going to medical school and then law school?

A: When I decided to go to medical school, everyone was supportive– of course. Then when I decided to go to law school, it was met with a lot more skepticism from pretty much everybody. One problem with saying you're interested in health policy is like saying you're interested in business or management, or those nebulous things that are conversation stoppers. People know what it is to be a doctor or a lawyer, but when you say "health policy," most people don't relate.

There weren't many people who thought it was a good idea. But, at that point, I'd pretty much made up my mind; I was just asking out of courtesy. And no one pushed back too much. They were supportive enough to accept my decision.

Q: Was there ever a time you wanted to give up?

A: One time I was talking to somebody who has this pristine pedigree; you know, multiple graduate degrees, all from Ivy League schools. I told her that was what I was interested in doing. She said, "That's great. But, there's no way you're going to be able to do it because you didn't go to the right schools. You went to Arizona State for law school and to Mayo for medical school and they're not Ivy League schools. It's very nice you're interested in this, but it's never going to go anywhere for you."

For maybe a day, that made me question a little bit: "Did I not think through this right? Am I going about this all wrong? Is this wasted time?"

But, I think I've been lucky to have a lot of good people around me who were pretty quick to jump on that and say, "I don't know what she's talking about. She hasn't met you."

Being able to share my insecurity from that conversation and have other people support me helped me get over that.

Since then, I've had other people tell me, "This is how you have to do it or you're not going to succeed." And what they're telling me to do is something I know I'm not going to do. But, since I've been told that so many times and they never seem to be right, I've gotten better at just kind of nodding and moving on. I've gotten a little less sensitive to peoples' skepticism and criticism.

Q: Is there anything that happened on your journey you didn't predict but proved to be valuable?

A: On one project I worked on, there was someone at the university I wanted to work with. He came up with an idea about reimbursement policy. It was something I knew nothing about, and had no real interest in. But, I really respected this person, and wanted to be able to work with him in the future. So, I said, "Okay, fine. I'll learn about this topic."

I spent the summer reading everything that had been written about it. I ended up writing a paper on it. Eventually, I knew as much as there was to know about this topic – kind of against my will.

When I ended up going to Washington and was called on to come up with innovative reimbursement policies for medical devices, the topic I worked on all summer happened to be the perfect background for that job. If I hadn't had that background, there's no way I could have done anything useful in that position. It was just pure luck. It worked out incredibly well for me, but I could never have predicted it.

Q: Looking back, is there anything you'd have done differently?

A: Professionally, even the things I ended up hating were good experiences. I had somebody tell me, "Never get involved with a research project you're not really interested in, because it will get so long and boring you'll regret it." I was too stubborn. People have given me lots of great advice I haven't followed.

I look at some of these experiences and realize I should have followed their advice – gotten interested in those research projects that were super boring and other super painful experiences. But, I don't regret doing them because that's how I have to learn. I make mistakes for myself. So, I don't know that I'd change much about what I've done in the past.

Q: What's been your greatest success or accomplishment?

A: The thing I'm most proud of started when I was in medical school. I worked at a free clinic in Rochester and started a prescription assistance program, aimed at getting free prescription drugs directly from the manufacturers for uninsured patients. Mayo, at the time, was funding the clinic to the tune of $300,000 a year, and every year we had to ask for new funding.

I wanted to start one of these programs and see if we could bring down the cost of the clinic a little bit so we didn't get cut off. Over about a three-month period, I was able to save about $60,000 of cost from patients just by filling out the applications with them and having them sent.

By good fortune, a few people from Pfizer came in and toured the clinic and the med school and wanted to see the free clinic. They reviewed the prescription assistance program and thought it was a good cause. They ended up saying, "Well, we have end of the year money we could give you, but we'd like to learn more about the patients who are using it. If so, we could help fund this study."

We ended up hiring someone to do what I'd been doing – filling out prescriptions for the patients. As a result, Pfizer agreed to fund a three-year study. By the end of the third year, we were saving Mayo directly about $700,000 a year and getting patients access to lots of medications they wouldn't have been able to have without the program.

The reason this is my greatest success is because there were so many moments of me banging my head against the wall pretty hard. It was incredibly frustrating, but in the end it worked out.

Q: What advice would you have for someone who wants to follow in your footsteps?

A: Learn to say, "No." At first, you seize every opportunity you can possibly get your hands on because you're a student and good chances may not come easily. But as you progress and gain experience, people will start asking you to become involved in things because you've developed a skill set or knowledge about them. It's hard to go from seeking opportunities for growth to learning how to say "no" to opportunities when they come.

It's definitely possible to get stretched too thin. At some point, everything has an increasing opportunity cost, and being able to prioritize and know it's okay to limit yourself to what you're interested in – not what everybody else is interested in – and to respect your own time and energy doesn't come naturally.

Also, recognize that there are so many smart people out there. Coming out of college, I wanted to learn law, medicine, economics, and every field I needed to know to be able to do everything I wanted. But, being able to have good people around you and recognize their expertise is incredibly important. I've learned more from people along the way than in the classroom and books. Keeping your mind open to the smart people around you will give you a lot more insight than you can get on your own. In the real world, almost everything worth doing requires a team of people with different skill sets; don't think you have to know and do everything by yourself.

Q: Would you recommend people go into medicine?

A: Yes – Yes – if you want to do it, go for it. It's worth spending some time to make sure you know what you're getting yourself into, but if you think you want to do it, just do it. What's the worst that could happen? You end up hating it and drop out? Fine – I guarantee you'll learn something along the way.

Q: What factors are most important in choosing a medical school?

A: The path to the medical field is pretty well mapped out for you. There's not a lot of flexibility there. You have to do all your undergraduate, pre-med classes. Then there are four years of medical school and then your training.

I once thought location was important in choosing a medical school. I finally realized it's not important at all because medical school will take up a lot of your time, and the curriculum is a lot more important than where you're living.

Also, it's important how they grade you in the first two years. At Mayo and a number of other schools, it's completely pass/fail; so, there are only two tiers of grading. Pretty much everyone passes. The reason that's important isn't that you want to go somewhere where you can slack off, but it shows you a lot about the administration's value system.

Schools that use traditional grading put a lot of pressure on students to be at the top of the class, and they take the emphasis off the importance of collaboration and teamwork. These are things that are important in the real world, but being in a system with traditional grading makes medical training a very individual experience. At a pass/fail school, it's that way intentionally because they want you to work together, they want you to have a work/life balance, and they don't want you to spend a lot of time worrying about the grade you're getting.

That's incredibly important for not only coming out of medical school with good mental health, good balance, and the ability to work with people; but it also gives you the opportunity to think about what you want to do with the rest of your life, and not just focus on winning the grading competition with your classmates.

Finally, schools that offer clinical exposure are valuable. My school had early clinical exposure, something I hadn't valued at all when I was choosing it. I was talking to friends at other schools who didn't get to see a real patient for the first two years. They forgot why they went into medicine and weren't sure they wanted to be in it anymore. When you just go through grueling schoolwork for two years and don't get to see any patients, you tend to lose your focus.

ACTION GUIDE

An easy reference guide to the advice and tips provided by Rachel Lindor

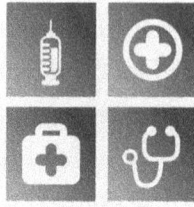

1) Learn to Say No!!!

One piece of advice people keep giving me, which I recognize is important, but I'm still bad at, is to learn to say, "No." I know people deal with that their whole lives. At some point, people may keep asking you to get involved in things because you've developed a skill set or knowledge about them. It's hard to go from seeking opportunities to learning how to say "No" to opportunities when they come. But, it's definitely possible to get stretched too thin.

2) Recognize the Importance of Teamwork

Teamwork is more important than you may realize when you're younger. You aren't going to accomplish anything meaningful on your own. Being able to have good people around you and recognize their expertise is important. I've learned more from the people I've met along the way than in the actual classroom and books. Keeping your mind open to the smart people around you will give you a lot of insight that you might not get otherwise.

3) Know What You're Looking For in a Medical School

I always thought location was important. Then I came to realize that it's not important at all because medical school will take up a lot of your time, and the curriculum is a lot more important than where you're living.

4) Don't be Intimidated by Medical School

Take the time to think about what you want to do in your career. People get intimidated by medical school. They think, "I just need to get through it and I'll be a doctor." But it would help to have an idea of what else you want to do beside seeing patients. In fact, most doctors do something else. They work in an institution and have other responsibilities – maybe administrative or educational or something. Knowing that going in is useful because you'll have time to think about it.

5) Start With the End in Sight

I was able to get a lot out of school because I always had an interest in policy. I encourage people to recognize that the end of the path doesn't have to just be being a doctor and seeing patients. You need to think about what else you want to do with your career.

CHAPTER 6

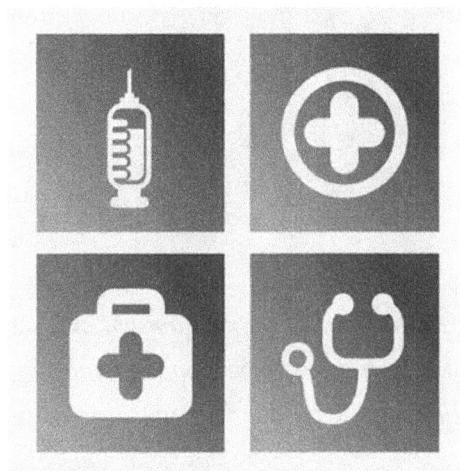

Dr. Angela Nuzzarello

BIOGRAPHY

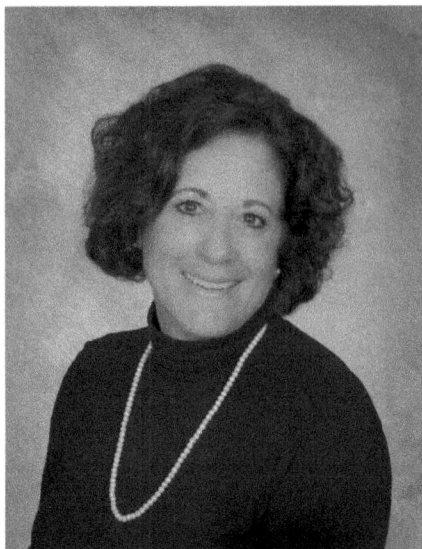

"I am not motivated by money, and I am not motivated by prestige and all that. I am motivated by passion – I really think that is what keeps me going. I have to wake up every morning to do this. I can't even imagine doing something other than what I'm passionate about."

– Dr. Angela Nuzzarello

Dr. Angela Nuzzarello is currently the Medical Director for Physician Wellness at Beaumont Health, an eight-hospital system in Southeast Michigan. She has spent almost 30 years in medical education and student affairs, focusing on the career development and wellness of medical students and physicians.

Dr. Nuzzarello graduated from Loyola University in Chicago with a Bachelor of Science degree in psychology. She then attended Rosalind Franklin University of Medicine and Science/Chicago Medical School and graduated in 1986. She served as Chief Resident in her psychiatry residency at Rush Presbyterian St. Luke's Medical Center and in 2003, she received a master's degree in health professions education from the University of Illinois College of Medicine at Chicago.

Dr. Nuzzarello's career in education began her first day of her first job, when her boss offered her the role of director of education for the Psychiatry Department at the University of Illinois College of Medicine at Peoria. A few years later, in 1993, she joined Northwestern University Feinberg School of Medicine, as Associate Professor in the Department of Psychiatry and Behavioral Sciences, and Assistant Professor in the Augusta Webster Office of Medical Education.

In 2004, Dr. Nuzzarello was appointed Associate Dean for Student Programs and Professional Development at Northwestern. In 2009, she was hired to build the Student Affairs program at a new medical school, Oakland University William Beaumont School of Medicine (OUWB). It was at OUWB that Dr. Nuzzarello developed and led a mentoring program with a curriculum focused on the personal development of medical students.

Dr. Nuzzarello has won numerous teaching awards throughout her educational career, including a Dean's Award for Teaching Excellence and four awards for Outstanding Basic Science Teacher. In 2015, she was awarded an Exceptional Mentor Award by the American Medical Women's Association for going above and beyond to actively guide those around her in their career paths.

INTERVIEW

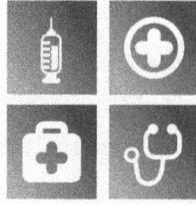

Q: Did you always want to be a doctor?

A: I wasn't one of those people who always knew I wanted to be a doctor. I started college in dental hygiene and I lasted about a day-and-a-half and realized right off the bat it wasn't going to be my path.

The reason I was looking into this dental hygiene program was that it was only a three-year program. I was dating a guy and thought I wanted to get through college quickly. Then, later in college, I decided, "You know, maybe I should try medical school." My dad, who was a physician and an old-fashioned guy, was saying, "There's no reason you shouldn't." So, that was how I ended up in medical school.

Q: Were you passionate about pediatrics?

A: I was doing research in child development when I was in college, and that sparked my interest. I love kids. I grew up around a lot of doctors. It wasn't like I pulled it out of the blue. I thought, "Oh, maybe I'd enjoy being a pediatrician." I had a lot of respect for them; I had a lot of respect for my dad.

Sometimes when I look back I think, "You know, I should have thought of it earlier." It seems an obvious thing. Why didn't I think of it sooner? I can't answer that.

Q: What did you do after medical school?

A: After medical school I did a residency in psychiatry. My career plan at that time was to be a psychiatrist and maybe work at a hospital and do some outpatient work. I got interested in the treatment of anxiety disorders.

The first day of my first job my boss came to me and said, "Just yesterday the person who was in charge of education for the department quit. So, would you be interested in taking on this role of director in charge of education in the department?"

It was my first day and I couldn't say, "I'm too busy." So, I said, "Of course." I had done a little teaching in my residency and enjoyed it. I was excited about it. When I look back, that was the start of my career because my career now is in education. But, that wasn't planned.

I did that for a while – a couple of years – and then a job opened up in education in psychiatry at Northwestern. I interviewed for the job and I got it. So the early part of my career was in education within psychiatry departments.

Q: How did you end up teaching in medical school?

A: When I got to Northwestern, my boss said, "You know, you should introduce yourself to people at the medical school." I made appointments with all of the deans – the Student Affairs Dean and the Education Dean and the Research Dean – and I went around and sat down individually and introduced myself.

I said, "I'm new here and this is what I'm interested in." I didn't know at the time that people didn't usually do that; but I didn't know any better. I remember when I was talking with the Student Affairs Dean, I thought, "Wow, that's a great job because he gets to really connect with the students and help those who are struggling, and I'm into building relationships and helping people. Maybe it would be a good match for me."

I ended up staying at Northwestern for 17 years, and then felt the need to make a change. I'd heard about a lot of new medical schools opening, and that appealed to my creative side. I love to create things and see things grow and nurture. So, I applied for this job at a new medical school and started there in January 2009.

Q: Is continuing education important?

A: Yes, it is. Part of what I love about my career is that I'm learning all sorts of new things because I teach. One of the reasons I took this job at a new medical school was for the opportunity to create a course in personal development for medical students.

Q: Was there ever a time you wanted to quit medical school?

A: Yes, I absolutely had moments where I thought I was in above my head. When I was in college, I studied psychology and philosophy. So, my exams were essay exams, and I liked talking about concepts and ideas. When I got into medical school, it was a lot of memorization. That wasn't my strong point. There were times when I thought, "I don't know if this is the best fit. I don't know if I can do this."

Q: Did you have a lot of support in medical school?

A: I had unbelievably awesome support. There was one dean in particular who was wonderfully supportive and was one of the most influential people in my life. I don't think it was any accident that I ended up as a Student Affairs dean, because when I think back to the times that were hard for me there was someone saying, "You can do this. I know you can do this!"

My brother was also supportive of me. We were in medical school together. He's a year older but we were in the same class. He has this attitude where he'd say, "You know what, Angela? You can do this. Don't let them get you down. Know what you have to do, and do it." He was a wonderful source of support for me, as was my entire family.

Q: Do you see a difference between someone who has a strong support group and somebody who doesn't?

Yes, I see a huge difference. Having that support makes all the difference. That's the biggest reason why I do what I do because I know how important that is. I feel I can be there for the students who maybe do have good support systems but I need to be there for those who don't. For those students who may be feeling lost, I can provide personal support but can also help them find professional help. I have even facilitated student to student support.

I've had so many times where students have said, "You know, I don't know if I would've made it if you haven't been there." That's what makes me feel fulfilled.

Q: Was passion important in the pursuit of your goals?

A: Passion, for me, was 90 percent of it. I don't know that I could continue to do what I'm doing without passion. It's hard; I have long days. I have three kids and a husband and a lot of other interests. It's passion that keeps me going when I think about this course I've developed and how I want to see that through.

I'm not motivated by money, and I'm not motivated by prestige and all that. I'm motivated by passion – that's what keeps me going.

Q: Should passion play a role in deciding on a career path?

A: You'll never be disappointed in what you're doing if you're passionate about it. You'll always love what you're doing. The reality of the situation, too, is that you know you've got to pay bills.

For medical students, there's a wide range of earning power, depending on what career path you choose. I could be making a lot more money if I was doing clinical practice instead of being in education. But, I'd never, ever tell a student to pursue something for money. You've got to wake up every morning to do this. I can't even imagine doing something other than what you're passionate about.

Q: What's your greatest success or accomplishment?

A: The first thing that comes to mind is being able to manage having a career and a family. To me, I feel good about the fact that I've been able to do both and be successful at both.

My biggest successes are the little things. One day, I was meeting with a student who was struggling. I told her that all of us at the medical school are behind her and that we believe she can be successful. She was accepted into medical school because we knew she had what it takes to succeed. She looked at me and said, "Oh, my gosh, Dr. Nuzzarello. All I needed to hear was that this was a doable thing and I'm able to do it."

Just the fact that I was able to connect and reach a student and maybe lighten her load a little bit is success. At the end of the day I felt good. I did what I was supposed to do, which was connect, reassure, and give someone some hope who felt like she couldn't do it.

Q: What was your greatest miscalculation?

A: On a daily basis, the thing I fail at most, and what I have to watch, is that I sometimes get overwhelmed. When that happens, I lose my focus. I lose who I am and what I need to do. So, I have to step back and refocus.

Also, I had a situation in a previous position where I was surrounded by people who were unsupportive and negative. I stayed in that environment a little too long, and finally I got to the point where I was feeling depleted. When I look back, I think, "Wow, I should have gotten myself out of that situation a lot faster." I didn't, so I see that as a failure.

Q: What make you happier, achievement itself, or the pursuit of it?

AI wouldn't say the pursuit. I'm always happy doing what I'm doing. But after I'm doing it for a while, I say to myself, "Hmm, what else can I do?" Maybe that's because I'm a creative person.

I'm drawn to creativity. All the people at work laugh at me because I'm always two steps ahead and thinking, "What could we do? What could be possible? What could we build? How could this be better? How could this be different?" I'm always thinking of a better way of doing things.

I recently met with a group of people and said, "I want to develop a wellness program. I want to get students involved and I want to hear from everybody how we can keep our focus on being well." That's the stuff I get crazy over and I love.

Creativity is important – at least to me. I had a position where creativity wasn't valued. It was pretty much, "Look, this is what needs to get done. You do it." So, getting things accomplished was valued, but new ideas weren't valued and creativity wasn't valued.

Part of my success was realizing what's important to me. It's not only being a good employee and doing what someone else thinks should be done, but looking deep inside and saying, "What makes me happy? What makes me feel alive? What fuels my passion?" A turning point in my career was realizing what's going to keep me going and what's going to keep me happy, and that was being able to nurture my creative spirit.

Q: If you had to do it again, what would you do differently?

A: I wouldn't change a whole lot. I could have gone in many different directions. Ultimately, I could have been happy doing a lot of different things. Sometimes I think, "Boy, it ends up that what I am is basically a teacher. Did I have to go through medical school and all of that?"

But then again, I don't think I'd be where I am if I didn't do it the way I did. I would've tried harder in college – probably 80 percent of the population say that. I don't know what I'd do differently. I've had a great ride. I like the fact that I didn't know all along where I'd end up.

I like that. It's not like I knew when I started out that this is what I was going to be doing.

Q: What advice would you give to those who want to follow in your footsteps?

A: The first piece of advice: Don't compromise. It goes back to this whole thing about if you're going to be successful you have to be who you are, and you can't compromise who you are or your values because you can't be successful in any environment.

Another bit of advice is to always do more than is expected of you. One of the reasons I was successful early on in my career was that I always did more than what was expected of me. If someone said, "I need you to work on this or do this." I'd do it and then I'd think, "Okay, what else? What could I do to make this a little bit different or a little bit better? You know, that extra push."

It's something I tell my kids all the time. Do what's expected, but do something else. It adds value, because people know if they give me something to do, something better is going to come out of it.

Also, appreciate the people who make you look good on a daily basis. Anybody who's successful has so many people around – whether it's family members or other people you work with. There are a lot of people who make me look good a lot of the time. It's important to make sure you appreciate those people and let them know how much value there is in what they do.

The last thing is about being dependable and trying to figure out how you can lighten someone else's load. That's always appreciated when you're not centered on yourself but you're also thinking about what you can do for someone else.

Q: What resources would you suggest for somebody who wishes to have a career like yours?

A: Spend a lot of time talking to people who are doing the work. Talk to people in different areas to see what might be a good fit for you, Ask what they like about their job and what they aren't so crazy about.

We do this with students, too, when trying to find out what specialty they want to go into. It's about finding out through questions what they like, what they don't like, how to get there. Also, I grew up around doctors, but a lot of people haven't. It's important to put yourself in that situation and see if it's the environment you'd feel comfortable in. That's important to do with medicine.

Specifically, if you want to go into medicine, it's more important to get involved in activities that allow you to be around people to see if that's where your talents lie. A lot of people say, "Oh, medicine. That sounds prestigious! Everybody will respect me." You know, those days are gone.

ACTION GUIDE

An easy reference guide to the advice and tips provided by Dr. Angela Nuzzarello

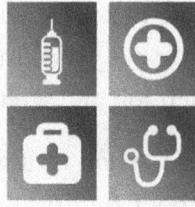

1) Don't Compromise

Don't compromise. If you're going to be successful you have to be who you are, and you can't compromise who you are or your values, because you can't be successful in any environment.

2) Always do More than Expected

Always do more than is expected of you. One of the reasons I was successful early on in my career was that I always did more than what was expected of me. If someone said, "I need you to work on this or do this." I'd do that and then I'd think, "Okay, what else? What could I do to make this a little bit different or a little bit better? You know, that extra push."

3) Appreciate the People Who Make You Look Good

Appreciate the people who make you look good on a daily basis. Anybody who's successful has so many people around – whether it's family members or other people you work with. There are a lot of people who make me look good a lot of the time. It's important to make sure you appreciate those people and let them know how much value there is in what they do.

4) Be Dependable

Be dependable and try to figure out how you can lighten someone else's load. That's always appreciated when you're not centered on yourself but you're also thinking about what you can do for someone else.

5) Talk to People Who are Already Doing the Work You Want to Do

Spend a lot of time talking to people who are doing the work. Student Affairs is the kind of thing where people don't generally plan a career. We all fall into it. But, it's important to talk to a lot of people who are doing that and find out.

RESOURCES

*A quick guide of helpful resources for
those aspiring in medicine*

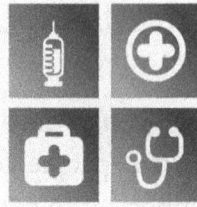

American Association of Family Physicians
www.aafp.org/about/the-aafp/vision.html

The American Academy of Family Physicians and its chapters proudly represent more than 115,900 family physician, resident, and medical student members. Family physicians play a critical role in improving the health of patients, families, and communities across the United States. The AAFP is committed to helping family physicians improve the health of Americans by advancing the specialty of family medicine, saving members' time, and maximizing the value of membership. Our focus every day is to help family physicians spend more time doing what they do best: providing quality and cost-effective patient care. The AAFP delivers value to its members through each of its strategic priorities.

American College of Emergency Physicians (ACEP)
www.acep.org

The American College of Emergency Physicians promotes the highest quality of emergency care and is the leading advocate for emergency physicians, their patients, and the public.

American College of Surgeons
www.facs.org/member-services/benefits/medical-student

Becoming a Medical Student Member of the American College of Surgeons (ACS) demonstrates your interest in a surgical career and a commitment to learn more about this exciting and challenging profession. The College is here to help you attain your professional goals and support you on your path to Fellowship.

American Medical Association
www.ama-assn.org/ama/home.page

As the nation's health care system continues to evolve, the AMA is dedicated to ensuring sustainable physician practices that result in better health outcomes for patients. This work is captured in the AMA's five-year strategic plan, which aims to ensure that enhancements to health care in the United States are physician-led, advance the physician-patient relationship, and ensure that health care costs can be prudently managed.

American Medical Women's Association (AMWA)
www.amwa-doc.org

AMWA membership is comprised of physicians, residents, medical students, and health care professionals. AMWA is the oldest multispecialty organization dedicated to advancing women in medicine and improving women's health.

American Society for Bariatric and Metabolic Surgery
https://asmbs.org/

After completing undergraduate, medical school and graduate medical education (GME), physicians still must obtain a license to practice medicine from a state or jurisdiction of the United States in which they are planning to practice. They apply for the permanent license after completing a series of exams and completing a minimum number of years of graduate medical education. The majority of physicians also choose to become board certified, which is an optional, voluntary process. Certification ensures that the doctor has been tested to assess his or her knowledge, skills, and experience in a specialty and is deemed qualified to provide quality patient care in that specialty. There are two levels of certification through 24 specialty medical boards — doctors can be certified in 36 general medical specialties and in an additional 88 subspecialty fields. Most certifications must be renewed after six to 10 years, depending on the specialty.

Army Medicine
www.goarmy.com/amedd/education.html

Whether you've just begun your undergraduate studies or have accepted a seat in medical school, you can take advantage of the programs the U.S. Army provides for students pursuing careers in health care. Our health care team consists of six corps, with more than 90 areas of concentration. Whatever the specialty, you'll have the opportunity to build a career of which you can be proud.

Association of American Medical Colleges
www.aamc.org/

Founded in 1876 and based in Washington, D.C., the Association of American Medical Colleges (AAMC) is a not-for-profit association representing all 141 accredited U.S. and 17 accredited Canadian medical schools; nearly 400 major teaching hospitals and health systems, including 51 Department of Veterans Affairs medical centers; and 90 academic and scientific societies. Through these institutions and organizations, the AAMC represents 128,000 faculty members, 83,000 medical students, and 110,000 resident physicians.

Association of Women Surgeons

www.womensurgeons.org/home/index.asp

The Association of Women Surgeons is committed to supporting the professional and personal needs of female surgeons at various stages in their careers – from residency through retirement. Since our founding in 1981, AWS has set up many programs with the specific objective of promoting the professional growth and advancement of our members.

Becoming a Pediatrician

www.aap.org/en-us/about-the-aap/Committees- Councils-Sections/Medical-Students/Pages/Becoming- A-Pediatrician.aspx

Becoming a Pediatrician: Your Guide to Exploring Pediatrics, Matching for Residency and Starting Intern Year is a publication meant to assist medical students who've already chosen pediatrics as a career. This resource will help you choose what electives to take in your fourth year of medical school, how to apply and interview for residency and finally how to be successful your first year of residency.

Being a Peace Corps Health Care Volunteer

www.peacecorps.gov/resources/faf/fafhealth/

The comprehensive medical evaluation in the second stage of the application process facilitates the placement of a Volunteer in a country that has adequate resources to meet the health care needs of the Volunteer. The Peace Corps staff includes at least one medical officer at each country's post. Nurses, nurse practitioners, physician assistants and physicians can serve as a Peace Corps medical officer. These dedicated providers include host-country nationals, third-country nationals and Americans. They are all carefully evaluated and credentialed by Peace Corps' Office of Medical Services Quality Improvement Unit at Headquarters. The quality of medical care at the posts is monitored regularly by the Office of Medical Services at Peace Corps headquarters.

Bureau of Labor and Statistics Occupational Outlook Handbook – Physicians and Surgeons
www.bls.gov/ooh/healthcare/physicians-and-surgeons.htm

Physicians and surgeons diagnose and treat injuries or illnesses. Physicians examine patients; take medical histories; prescribe medications; and order, perform, and interpret diagnostic tests. They counsel patients on diet, hygiene, and preventive healthcare. Surgeons operate on patients to treat injuries, such as broken bones; diseases, such as cancerous tumors; and deformities, such as cleft palates. Physicians and surgeons held about 691,400 jobs in 2012.

Many physicians work in private offices or clinics, often with administrative and healthcare personnel. Wages for physicians and surgeons are among the highest of all occupations. According to the Medical Group Management Association's Physician Compensation and Production Survey, median total compensation for physicians varied with their type of practice. In 2012, physicians practicing primary care received total median annual compensation of $220,942 and physicians practicing in medical specialties received total median annual compensation of $396,233.

Career Options for Doctors from AAMC
www.aamc.org/students/aspiring/career

Explore your medical career options. Read the "Aspiring Doc Diaries," watch the "Ask a Med Student" series. Find training opportunities for pre-med students.

Doctor Mentoring Resources
www.aafp.org/medical-school-residency/medical-school/mentoring.html

For medical students, having a physician who serves as a mentor may be one of the most valuable resources on the path to becoming a doctor. Mentoring relationships are particularly important for minority students or students who are in a medical school that does have a department of family medicine. Mentoring happens in both formal and informal settings. Some schools offer formal mentoring programs, special projects, or networking. More informal mechanisms may include leadership opportunities and special interest mentoring. Finding a family physician mentor in any of these categories may help in your path through school.

Join a Family Medicine Interest Group
www.aafp.org/medical-school-residency/fmig/connect.html

The AAFP established the National FMIG Network to aid communication and the exchange of best practices between FMIG students and faculty leaders across the country. The network consists of campus-based faculty and student FMIG leaders, appointed Regional Coordinators, and one elected National Coordinator. These coordinators serve as consultants to and resources for FMIGs.

Massachusetts Medical Society- Private Practice Ownership and Operations
www.massmed.org/Physicians/Practice-Management/Practice-Ownership-and-Operations/Practice- Ownership-and-Operations/#.VTgIShdvk2t

Resources here run the gamut from practice start-up tips and best practices for hiring staff to patient satisfaction surveys and locating discounted office supplies.

Mayo Medical School
www.mayo.edu/mms/

As a Mayo medical student, you are a respected member of a world-class health care team and will obtain the skills necessary to become a successful, fulfilled healer and health advocate as evidenced by the success of our students.

Medical College Admissions Test (MCAT)
www.aamc.org/students/applying/mcat/

This standardized, multiple-choice examination is designed to assess the examinee's problem solving, critical thinking, and knowledge of science concepts and principles prerequisite to the study of medicine. Scores are reported in Physical Sciences, Verbal Reasoning, and Biological Sciences. Almost all U.S. medical schools and many Canadian schools require applicants to submit MCAT exam scores. Many schools do not accept MCAT exam scores that are more than three years old.

Northwestern University Feinberg School of Medicine
www.feinberg.northwestern.edu/

A career in medicine offers a diverse range of opportunities to serve people in need. Medical schools are looking for bright and hard-working people who understand the needs of their communities and want to make a difference in the lives of others. If you're drawn to helping people and have the desire to use science and humanity to serve society, then a career in medicine might be the right choice for you.

Oakland University William Beaumont School of Medicine
www.oakland.edu/medicine

The Oakland University William Beaumont School of Medicine is a collaborative, diverse, inclusive, and technologically advanced learning community, dedicated to enabling students to become skillful, ethical, and compassionate physicians, inquisitive scientists invested in the scholarship of discovery, and dynamic and effective medical educators.

Practice Management Resources: American College of Physicians (ACP)

www.acponline.org/running_practice/practice_ management/

ACP and the Medical Group Management Association (MGMA) have collaborated to provide physicians with a landing page that pulls together shared MGMA and ACP practice management resources. Find resources on Your Medical Practice, Coding and Billing, Payer Relations, Patient Care Delivery, Practice Solution for Physicians, and Risk Management, Compliance and health policy.

Practice Management Resources from AAFP:

www.aafp.org/practice-management.html

For medical students, having a physician who serves as a mentor may be one of the most valuable resources on the path to becoming a doctor. Mentoring relationships are particularly important for minority students or students who are in a medical school that does have a department of family medicine. Mentoring happens in both formal and informal settings. Some schools offer formal mentoring programs, special projects, or networking. More informal mechanisms may include leadership opportunities and special interest mentoring. Finding a family physician mentor in any of these categories may help in your path through school.

Requirements for Becoming a Physician

www.ama-assn.org/ama/pub/education-careers/
becoming-physician

After completing undergraduate, medical school and graduate medical education (GME), physicians still must obtain a license to practice medicine from a state or jurisdiction of the United States in which they are planning to practice. They apply for the permanent license after completing a series of exams and completing a minimum number of years of graduate medical education. The majority of physicians also choose to become board certified, which is an optional, voluntary process. Certification ensures that the doctor has been tested to assess his or her knowledge, skills, and experience in a specialty and is deemed qualified to provide quality patient care in that specialty. There are two levels of certification through 24 specialty medical boards — doctors can be certified in 36 general medical specialties and in an additional 88 subspecialty fields. Most certifications must be renewed after six to 10 years, depending on the specialty.

Running your Business Like a Business - AAFP
www.aafp.org/fpm/2013/0900/p18.html

This medical practice uses technology and automaker-inspired productivity steps to modernize and rapidly grow your business.

Shufeldt Consulting
www.shufeldtconsulting.com/

The changing face of healthcare demands a diverse skill set to successfully manage a healthcare practice. Macroeconomic forces and increased governmental and insurance regulations have forced physicians and practice managers to be experts in a variety of fields while at the same time providing prompt, quality healthcare to their patients. Shufeldt Consulting provides professional consulting services to urgent care and medical office practices throughout the United States.

Student Doctor Network
www.studentdoctor.net/about-sdn/

We are a vibrant non-profit organization of thousands of pre-health, health professional students and practicing doctors from across the United States and Canada. Membership is free. The educational mission of SDN is to assist and encourage all students through the challenging and complicated healthcare education process and into practice. Our members have created one of the most active and supportive communities on the Internet, with many members making lifelong friendships. Many of our members started as undergraduates and are now practicing doctors in every field of medicine and healthcare. With tens of thousands of active members and millions of posts, our members can answer practically any question you may have, from college through advanced practice.

UC Davis: On Becoming a Doctor:
www.ucdmc.ucdavis.edu/mdprogram/admissions/ whyucdavis/ doctor.html

A career in medicine offers a diverse range of opportunities to serve people in need. Medical schools are looking for bright and hard-working people who understand the needs of their communities and want to make a difference in the lives of others. If you're drawn to helping people and have the desire to use science and humanity to serve society, then a career in medicine might be the right choice for you.

University of Colorado – General Surgery Residency
ucdenver.edu/academics/colleges/

medicalschool/departments/surgery/education/

GeneralSurgeryResidency/Pages/GeneralInformation.aspx

We offer a five-year, non-pyramidal general surgical residency training program, approved for 77 resident positions and to graduate ten chief residents in general surgery each year. The internship has thirty positions: ten categorical general surgery residents and eighteen preliminary positions in general surgery for individuals preparing for a residency in another discipline. The final two positions are Urology preliminary positions. There are also five preliminary positions available for a second clinical year of surgical training.

University of Texas Health Science Center in San Antonio
som.uthscsa.edu

A strong and supportive faculty, numerous opportunities for building clinical and research skills, and a high quality of life in a growing, prosperous city are a few of the reasons that distinguish us. Located in the heart of the South Texas Medical Center, we are a major part of the health care and bioscience industry of the area, and we have a firm commitment to serve the communities within San Antonio and the surrounding region.

Wayne State University School of Medicine
admissions.med.wayne.edu/

The Wayne State University SOM Office of Admissions is committed to providing a first-rate medical education for our medical students. With our long standing commitment to education, research and patient care, we aim to make the admissions process with the School of Medicine as straight-forward and smooth as possible.

World Health Organization
www.who.int/topics/health_policy/en

Health policy refers to decisions, plans, and actions that are undertaken to achieve specific health care goals within a society. An explicit health policy can achieve several things: it defines a vision for the future which in turn helps to establish targets and points of reference for the short and medium term. It outlines priorities and the expected roles of different groups; and it builds consensus and informs people.

CONCLUSION

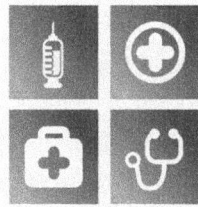

It's my sincere hope that these amazing outliers motivate you as much as they did me. Their stories reveal what may not have been apparent from the perspective of an outsider, who may have thought that, given their successes, their paths were straight and easy. To hear their stories about how they faced setbacks and adapted to adversity, told in such an honest and straightforward manner, is both sobering and inspiring.

What is so transparent is that none of these individuals had anything simply handed to them. They all fought hard for their accomplishments and were ultimately successful through perseverance, humility and by following their passion. They were not perfect nor were they on a straight trajectory. No one is.

What their stories illustrate is that all of us can aspire to greatness and accomplish anything we're passionate about, as long as we persevere and accept some failures along the way. Maybe after passion, the most important attribute is to be fearless as it relates to failure. In other words, accept the fact that you'll likely fail your way to success because, at the end of the day – if it were easy, everyone would do it, and success would be no accomplishment at all.

The Action Guides offer step-by-step outlines from each outlier on a potential path to success, and the Resource Guides will provide additional sources of information.

You now have everything you need: six great mentors, a path to follow, and some additional resources to help you along the way. What are you waiting for? Go out and accomplish your most amazing future, and join the ranks of the outliers!

I'll end this as I've ended the other books in the series with a quote from Mark Twain:

Twenty years from now you will be more disappointed by the things that you didn't do than by the ones you did do. So throw off the bowlines. Sail away from the safe harbor. Catch the trade winds in your sails.

Explore. Dream. Discover.

FOLLOW THE OUTLIER MOVEMENT

www.facebook.com/readingredientsofoutliers

www.twitter.com/JohnShufeldt

ingredientsofoutliers@gmail.com

ADDITIONAL WORKS
BY DR. JOHN SHUFELDT

The Outlier Series

Ingredients of Outliers: A Recipe for Personal Achievement
June 2013

Ingredients of Young Outliers: Achieving Your Most Amazing Future
March 2014

Ingredients of Outliers: Women Game Changers
January 2015

Outliers in Medicine
April 2015

LeadershipYOU: Your Future Starts With You
April 2017

You Economy: Inspiring Your Inner Entrepreneur
March 2018

Upcoming Works

Dr. Shufeldt is currently writing the rest of the Outlier Series, which will include career-specific books featuring exceptional individuals he calls "outliers." The books in the series will introduce students or prospective professionals in several fields of interest to the insider tips on becoming an outlier in their respective profession. Upcoming titles include:

Outliers in Law

www.ingramcontent.com/pod-product-compliance
Lightning Source LLC
Chambersburg PA
CBHW071614040426
42452CB00008B/1338